MW01142051

Living Beside

PERFORMING NORMAL
AFTER INCEST MEMORIES RETURN

Tanya Lewis

an
all-girl production
from

McGILLIGAN
BOOKS

Canadian Cataloguing in Publication Data
Lewis, Tanya
  Living beside: performing normal after incest memories return

Includes bibliographical references.
ISBN 0-9698064-7-7

1. Incest victims - Mental health. 2. Lewis, Tanya - Mental health. 3. Psychotherapy. 4.
Recovered memory. I. Title.

RC560.I53L48 1999   616.85'8369   C99-930703-7

Copyright © Tanya Lewis 1999

Editor: Ann Decter
Copy editor: Noreen Shanahan
Layout: Denise Maxwell
Cover Design: Heather Guylar
Author Photo: Lewis

All rights reserved. No part of this book may be reproduced in any manner whatsoever
without written permission, except in the case of brief quotations in critical articles or
reviews. For information contact McGilligan Books, P.O. Box 16024, 859 Dundas Street
West, Toronto, ON, Canada, M6J 1W0, ph (416)538-0945, e-mail mcgilbks@idirect.com.

Contents

Chapter 1

BUMPING INTO NORMATIVITY

So he wrote it ... again and again as he ongoingly
glimpsed it and lost it.
C. WHITNEY-BROWN, 1996

Though nothing can bring back the hour
Of splendour in the grass, of glory in the flower;
We will grieve not, rather find
Strength in what remains behind.
WILLIAM WORDSWORTH

I remember weeping uncontrollably when I heard these words as a young teenager. They sounded a death knell, touching something I knew was true and could not recall.

As you read, remember that this writing was born of grief, confusion, anger and intuition. Clarity and linearity has been gained on a convoluted journey over time and experience, held by a flicker of stubborn hope within despair.

Eleven years ago, when I was thirty-five, I recovered my first memories of incest as a child. I was married, at the time, with two young children and completing a Master's degree. As my world was opening up intellectually, emotionally I felt as if I had come to a dead end. Everything I knew how to do, to help myself feel better and to cope, no longer worked. The return of incest memories had an impact on every aspect of my life. The process, as I experienced it, was a bit like landing on a desert island resembling a shell of my former home. The effectiveness of the survival strategies I used in the past to negotiate the world were slowly and systematically being cut away through the therapeutic process. How was I to live? Increasingly less

1

numb, physically and emotionally, less able to escape relationships through dissociation, how was I to survive?

With the return of memories that rocked the assumptions through which I had constructed my life – loyalty and fidelity to family – what was I to believe? What have incest memories taught me about the world and my place in it? How could I make sense of my struggles? On a pragmatic level, how would I spend family holidays? Responding to these shifts, intellectually, emotionally and physically fundamentally altered my perspectives and priorities, and taught me much about how normative discourses frame my life and sense of myself.

The challenge I, like other trauma survivors, face is that "the moral function of memory is to compel us to confront what we – and all around us – wish to leave behind"(Kirmayer, 1996:193). Within therapeutic incest literature, this confrontation has been predominantly constructed in individual terms and focussed on recovering the forgotten past and on changing dysfunctional behaviour patterns of the survivor in the present (Bass & Davis, 1988). This psychological approach is inadequate. The confrontation the survivor faces daily is with discourses of normativity[1] which position her as "other" and maintain dominant forms of social power and privilege.

The concept of normative discourse refers to the shaping of individual identity through dominant systems of knowledge and power. Epstein and Johnson describe the concept of discourse saying:

> Human agents cannot stand outside culture and wield power precisely as they wish. Power is always limited and shaped by systems of knowledge which also shape the subjects and objects of power ... forms of power/knowledge position us as subjects of various kinds. They put pressure on us to adopt particular identities ... [and shape] fantasies of desire, enjoyment, fear, hatred, recognition, power and powerlessness. (1997: 15)

Individuals are thus shaped by and come to shape themselves in complex interactions with normative discourses. Normative discourses present idealized and particular portraits of how individuals are to conduct their lives. For example, affluent and affectionate heterosexual families, and employment in which talents and skills are maximized. In this sense, normative discourses regulate the formation and expression of desire, expectations, and behaviour. The goal for an individual becomes one of meeting dominant expectations and standards of performance to attain a life reflecting dominant ideals.

I take normativity to mean the everyday ways in which our desires, actions and behaviour are structured through "common sense" ideas of a "normal" that is constituted through normative discourses. It refers to the beliefs and practices which establish the regulatory dichotomy of "normal" and "other". Regardless of individual positioning within normative discourses, the work becomes one of maintaining one's stance as normal rather than other. The dichotomy of normal and other underlying normativity becomes a contested site of regulation and change. Deborah Britzman describes the primary site of this struggle:

> The production of normalcy, as Foucault points out is not 'a history of mentalities' or one of meaning, but rather a 'history of bodies' and hence the problem of how sociality can be lived and how politics can be imagined. (1998:85)

My awareness of how my life is constructed in and through discourses of normativity grew out of the process of recovering memory held in my body. Because repressed memory can be understood as a letting go of the defenses of denial and minimization, holding onto as much of my experience as possible depends on my capacity to not engage in denial. As I shifted my participation in discursive practices by letting my denial go, my awareness of how discourses of normativity maintain social patterns of power and privilege began to emerge intuitively. I frequently experienced this as divisive guilt-ridden splits between what I was expected to do and what holding onto emerging memory meant that I could not do. It has taken a long time for this knowledge to be articulated conceptually.

Why do I feel different from others? What am I responsible for and to whom? For most of my life I have lived with a sense of being different from others. While this was true before the return of incest memories, it continues to be my experience. As the therapeutic literature suggests, this sense of difference has lessened as I have loosened some of my self-blame for my abuse and strengthened my self-acceptance (Herman, 1992). However, the positioning of incest as "other", different from the norm, creates and maintains my life experiences as different from those of others.

Because I am frequently reluctant to embrace the ways therapeutic literature states I can help myself, my sense of difference is reinforced. In exploring the complexity underlying my reluctance, the importance of discourses of normativity in framing my everyday life has come to the forefront.

Denial is a fundamental mechanism for surviving abuse. Now, maintaining my sense of self depends on not engaging in denial, not numbing my body, rationalizing my feelings or dissociating. As I engage less in denial, my awareness of its broad role in maintaining everyday life for everyone is enhanced, leaving me feeling different once again. Living with this ongoing experience of difference, I seem to be in a constant internal conversation with discourses of normativity. This conversation has clarified how an incest survivor's experience is constructed through the frame of "normal".

The question of what I am responsible for in life and to whom can be partially understood in therapeutic terms as confronting the legacies of incest: the disproportionate amount of caretaking and blame I assume in relationships (Bass & Davis, 1988). My struggle to establish appropriate boundaries in relationships and to break my denial regarding my past led to very different relationships with family members, some of whom were aging and have since died. During therapy, I became very aware of the power normative discourses surrounding family had within my own life and lives of others. At the same time, to follow the recommendations of therapeutic discourses to establish relationships with family members on my terms felt insensitive to those whose lives were ending. Sitting between a rock and a hard place, I developed insight into the relationship between two prescriptive systems of thought and behaviour, therapeutic discourses and discourses of normativity.

The question of responsibility is also driven by my desire not to participate in practices of domination which lead to violence against women and children. Although the therapeutic incest literature absolves me of responsibility for the incest based on the power differentials between an adult and a child (Bass & Davis, 1988), as an adult survivor I am responsible for the choices I make, for what I reproduce from the past and refuse in the present[2]. Not living in denial means I am more aware of my responsibility. And, living with the legacies of incest, terror and fear of annihilation, adds a layer of physical and emotional complexity to my desire to work for change.

In her exploration of trauma literatures about Vietnam war veterans, holocaust and incest survivors, Kali Tal pinpoints the survivors struggle and desire for change:

> Bearing witness is an aggressive act. It is born out of a refusal to
> bow to outside pressure to revise or repress experience, a deci-

sion to embrace conflict rather than conformity, to endure a lifetime of anger and pain rather than submit to the seductive pull of revision and repression. Its goal is change.(1996:7).

While I share this desire for change with other survivors, I am uncertain about what constitutes change. Even with all the work to increase the visibility of incest and to develop effective social responses, children are not protected from violation. Individual therapy, not social confrontation, predominates as the site of change (Armstrong, 1994).

Framing Incest
Kali Tal discusses how discourses of normativity frame traumatic experience to contain their disruptive potential. These frameworks are:

> . . . mythologization [which] works by reducing the traumatic event to a set of standardized narratives . . . turning it from a frightening and uncontrollable event into a contained and predictable narrative. Medicalization focuses our attention upon the victims of trauma, positing that they suffer from an "illness" that can be "cured" within existing or slightly modified structures of institutionalized medicine and psychiatry. Disappearance – a refusal to admit the existence of a particular kind of trauma – is usually accomplished by undermining the credibility of the victim.(1996:6)

These discourses of normativity have an impact on how incest is understood; none of them address the complexity of the questions I live with as an adult incest survivor.

Through the work of feminists over the past twenty-five years, incest has gained visibility and its victims have attained some measure of credibility in North America. Childhood sexual abuse has had an intermittent history of social visibility and invisibility as a problem (Herman, 1992). With the 'second wave' of feminism – beginning in the 1960s – women began speaking of their experiences of growing up in heterosexual families. At present, there is some social acknowledgement that childhood sexual abuse is part of many girl's experience and of the women they become.

The struggle for credibility, built through institutional support for research, required and created a standard narrative, what Tal refers to as mythologization. Defining the problem, studying its extent, and generating theories about its existence and prevalence became the focus. This process contains the horror of a child being raped within her family in existing frameworks of knowledge generation and response mechanisms.

In her study, *The Conspiracy of Silence,* Sandra Butler defines incest as:

> . . . any manual, oral, or genital sexual contact or other explicit sexual behaviour that an adult family member imposes on a child who is unable to alter or understand the adult's behaviour because of his or her powerlessness in the family and early stage of psychological development. (1985:4,5)

Almost fifteen years later, Health & Welfare Canada also recognizes the difference between adults who have power and children who don't as a distinguishing feature of abuse within their definition. Abuse is delineated as actions which result in injury or harm, physical, emotional, sexual or a combination of these. The harm which results from sexual abuse is identified as: difficulties maintaining regular body patterns of sleep and eating; struggling with trust, sexuality, depression, despair, fear, anxiety, slashing, flashbacks and unconscious reenactments of the traumatic event (Herman, 1992; Bass & Davis, 1988). Survivor's risk of revictimization through rape, battering and sexual harassment is double that of other women (Herman, 1992).

Several studies which examine the prevalence of childhood sexual abuse have also been completed. Judy Steed (1994) refers to the Canadian government's 1984 *Badgely Report* which concluded that one in four girls and one in seven boys experienced unwanted sexual acts. Steed also references a 1992 York University study in which 43% of females reported a sexual abuse experience in childhood, and 17% were incest survivors. Diane Russell's early work found one in three women had been sexually abused in childhood, 16% were incest survivors (Russell, 1986). These figures are regarded as conservative (Steed, 1994).

Theories which explain the existence and prevalence of childhood sexual abuse include perspectives from different academic disciplines. They can be separated into three streams of inquiry: psychological, sociological and feminist. Psychological explanations locate the source of the problem within individual pathology (Elliot, 1996). Characteristics of perpetrators which create a potential for abuse include poor self-esteem, substance abuse, rigid and controlling behaviour, severe communication problems in relationships and unrealistic expectations. Marital problems, financial difficulties and unemployment are seen as contributing factors (Sykes &

Symons-Moulton, 1991). Most of these theories focus on the personality development of the perpetrator in early childhood, though some look at biological, chemical and neurological disorders (Elliot, 1996). A subset of these psychological theories are interactional/systems models which emphasize the "dysfunction" of the family dynamics as setting the stage for incest (Forward & Buck, 1988). Emotional distance and confusion of roles and boundaries are seen as key factors. Underlying this emphasis on family "dysfunction" is the assumption that the "normal" family has the capacity to meet the needs of its members (Elliot, 1996).

Sociological perspectives examine the social structure of the family unit, as well as factors which create family stress. These include the private nature of family life, which makes detection of violence difficult, and the effects of social relations of power and labour within families. Characteristics examined include how roles and responsibilities are assigned by age and sex, rather than by competence or interest, the dependence of children on their family and the high degree of interaction among people who may have very different interests (Elliot, 1996). Other factors include social condoning of violence, and a social environment which does not provide adequate support for parents, such as poverty, isolation and poor housing (Elliot, 1996).

Feminist perspectives highlight how differences in power between men, women and children are played out in the "private" sphere of the family home (Butler, 1985; Armstrong, 1994). The social and economic power men have over women and children, as well as the construction of female gender as an object of male desire are seen as key factors contributing to childhood sexual abuse (Armstrong, 1994; Jacobs, 1993).

Theories frequently combine elements from these different perspectives, all of which agree that childhood sexual abuse involves an adult who desires sexual contact with a child (Sink, 1988). Steed (1994) understands this sexual contact as a way to feel powerful through sexually dominating children. Other writers like Jean Renvoize (1993) and Sandra Butler (1985) highlight the appearance of respectability of many families in which incest occurs and the tyranny with which the father rules the household. In such households, wives and mothers tend to live according to traditional sexual roles and are frequently economically dependent and disempowered. Describing the characteristics of mothers of incest survivors, Judith Lewis Herman (1993) highlights the frequency (approximately 50%) of chronic illness requiring hospitalization among mothers of incest survivors. Because of threats by the male family member over the child, and the lack of economic and emotional support the mother may have received, silence and denial prevailed.

Responses to Childhood Sexual Abuse

In addition to theorizing the problem of childhood sexual abuse, the purpose of research is to identify effective response mechanisms. These include intervention by child protection authorities as well as by the criminal justice system.

Mandatory reporting requirements of childhood sexual abuse designate responsibility for resolution. Wachtel (1989) outlines how the focus of intervention is on maintaining the family unit and protecting the child, if necessary through placement in care with child welfare agencies. Gunn & Linden (1994) found that approximately half the children in their study were placed in care. Sykes & Symons-Moulton (1991) summarize decisions regarding placement in care by saying "typically, however, every attempt will be made to provide treatment that is aimed at keeping families together or re-uniting them as soon as it is feasible and safe to do so" (141)[3].

The 1988 changes to the *Criminal Code* and the *Canada Evidence Act* create greater accommodation for children (Steed, 1994). However, prosecution is still difficult. Gunn & Linden (1994) found that the police considered physical evidence and the credibility of the complainant primary in laying charges. The ability of the child to testify under oath, the age of the child and corroborating witnesses are also important factors. However, because of the privatized nature of the offence, there are unlikely to be witnesses or evidence, and depending on their age, children may not make very credible witnesses. Armstrong (1994) outlines how women who try to defend their children through the courts frequently become objects of attack as the defence's focusses on destroying the mother's and children's credibility.

Legal interventions are also a possible route for adult survivors. Burstow cautions therapists to advise their clients to weigh the benefits and risks of legal action carefully. The result may be further empowerment, reduction of risk for the survivor and others, as well as financial remuneration; or the claim may be dismissed, the survivor may experience revictimization and possible threat from the perpetrator. Substantial documentation by the therapist is important and claims involving bodily harm are more likely to be successful than those involving psychological harm (1992:144). Herman cites that the reporting rate for sexual assaults on children is low (2-6%) and that "perpetrators are aided by the widespread bias against women that still pervades our [American] system of justice"(1996:13).

Social response through legal prosecution and child protection depends on demonstrating the legitimacy of the claim. Because questions of legitimacy are woven through the social fabric of power and privilege, this criteria contains little guarantee of an effective response from the point of view of the individual making the disclosure. While this point will be discussed further, what is guaranteed by disclosure is that the survivor will be viewed as requiring therapy. Discourses of medicalization are dominant (Tal, 1996).

Within discourses of medicalization, clients undergo a recovery process in which their trauma is dealt with by moving through predictable linear stages (Herman, 1992). Armstrong (1994) outlines the recent burgeoning of professionals offering one-on-one therapy, group work and self-help resources for survivors undergoing this recovery process within North America. The availability of therapeutic resources varies according to a woman's financial resources.

Most therapeutic approaches understand the survivor's task as one of resuming "normal" life as soon as possible (Herman, 1992). Many vary in their approach according to their underlying theoretical analysis. Some approaches focus on "dysfunctional" family dynamics, while others explore multiple personality disorder or utilize feminist critiques of male power and privilege. With the exception of Burstow (1992), Butler (1992) and Brown (1995), feminists who begin their writing with accounts of incest as being part of systemic male violence, usually end with the response of alleviating symptoms of violence through therapeutic help. The fact that recovery occurs within conditions of violence appears to be forgotten by most authors, including feminists.

The impact of these discourses in shaping how survivors' experience is perceived can not be underestimated. Change has become focussed on individual therapeutic healing rather than on the social and political shifts desired by the women who first spoke out about their incest experiences (Alcoff & Gray, 1993; Armstrong, 1994; Tal, 1996). While the development of a survivor mission is seen as part of the "recovery" process (Herman, 1992), it remains an individual rather than a social project. This medicalization of traumatic experience maintains social relations of power and privilege through individualizing and privatizing the site of the problem and its solution.

Discourses of Disappearance
Discourses of disappearance work less subtly than those of medicalization and mythologization. Using normative standards of legitimacy, these dis-

courses directly attack the credibility of survivors' experiences. This is not a recent phenomenon. Herman describes the "episodic amnesia" which has historically surrounded the visibility of trauma (1992:7). Freud's recanting of his seduction theory, in which children are initiated into adult sexuality, in favour of his oedipal theory, which reframes these experiences as the child's sexual fantasies, is a famous example of such episodic amnesia (Champagne, 1996).

The rise of the False Memory Syndrome Foundation over the past few years represents the clearest example of efforts to ignore trauma and discredit those who break silence. The False Memory Syndrome Foundation, begun by parents whose adult daughter accused her father of sexual abuse, questions the extent to which recovery of memory is possible and is influenced through suggestion by therapists or by reading self-help resources (Wakefield & Underwager; Backus & Stannard, 1994). Strategies used to cast doubt about the legitimacy of recovered memory include disbelief that respectable adults would molest children, questions regarding the harm of childhood sexual abuse and analogies between those who accuse perpetrators and witch hunts (Freyd, 1996).

Others contest these discourses of disappearance. In her review of current knowledge regarding the storage of traumatic memory, Judith Lewis Herman cites clinical work, an extensive literature review and studies which examine the verification of memories. She concludes that traumatic memory is focussed accurately on the main events and sensory detail, and is inaccurate with regard to time sequencing, context and peripheral detail (1996: 7,10). Research into the biochemistry of memory supports therapeutic claims of repressed memory (Van Der Kolk & Van Der Hart, 1995; Van Der Kolk, 1994). In her work on the role of betrayal in repressed memory, Jennifer Freyd examines existing studies to support her hypothesis that "repressed memory is higher in incest than in other forms of sexual abuse" (1996: 141). Through these on-going debates, strategies of disappearance divert energy and attention away from systemic change and into defending questions of legitimacy.

Defining Normal

The frameworks through which incest is understood and categorized by discourses of mythologization and medicalization, and by the questions of legitimacy raised in discourses of disappearance and intervention mechanisms reveal what can be referred to as the normative standards underlying social regulation of incest. These discourses implicitly pivot on definitions of "normal" experience based on positivist scientific methodology and on reestablishing the normal condition through social or individual intervention. Michel Foucault articulates how social regulation based on "normal" experience operates. Disciplinary practices compare, differentiate, hierarchize, homogenize and exclude human behaviour based on normative expectations (in Rabinow, 1984:195). The underlying punitive nature of these disciplinary practices can be seen in the labels assigned to those who live outside the boundaries: "mad" or as "sexual perverts" (145). By comparing an incest survivor's story to that of other "normal" adults and then differentiating it, the story remains that of an individual even if there are many individuals with the same or similar stories. The process of comparison and differentiation establishes a hierarchy between "normal" and "abnormal" experience.

Comparison to a "norm" also excludes contextual information that could develop a complex analysis of social relations of power and privilege (Kadi, 1996). For example, assigning merit for students based strictly on a comparison of knowledge and performance on marks, rather than on a consideration of other responsibilities for child care, access to financial support, sources of information, cultural differences maintains the privilege of those closest to the social ideal.

The scientific method, with its assertion of rational thought, natural processes and a preoccupation with the individual, is essential to developing and reinforcing these standards. Discovering normative standards of behaviour and functions, then measuring and reducing deviations from norms takes place within objective scientific frameworks. It is both descriptive of normative standards and capable of evaluating those who (do not) meet them (Venn, 1984; Hacking, 1996). Adherence to norms become the way in which individuals are seen to contribute to the social good (Venn, 1984: 146).

Psychology has played a major role in defining the realms of normal and abnormal behaviour. Paula Caplan outlines the criteria through which normalcy is defined within human behaviour. These definitions include infrequency or an absence of most conflict or anxiety. Also, because it defines clear developmental stages, psychology establishes abnormality as a delay or a fixation at a particular stage. Other criteria through which normal is defined include the need to test reality, too much, too little, or a lack of particular desirable behaviours (1995: 46-52).

Feminists have challenged scientific method as biased in favour of male gender experience and not reflective of women's experience and oppression.

Feminist work illustrates how male rule is constructed through control over resources, and through normative ideologies and social practices which foreground male experience as human and create female experience as "other" (Smith, 1987; Flax, 1986). For example, attributes considered to be male – such as mastery, rationality, control and autonomy – constitute the public domain, while attributes considered to be female – such as emotion, embodiment, relationality and care – are marginalized and relegated to the private domain (Benjamin, 1988).

What is interesting about the scientific construction of normal human behaviour is that it erases social power and privilege embedded in culture and history, and lived out in class, race and gender relations. Attaining social norms is positioned as the goal of human behaviour. Those who fail to do so are positioned as "other", diagnosed and taught skills through therapeutic intervention to overcome their "deficiencies", without any acknowledgement of social power and privilege. In describing the effects of such interventions on women, Chesler (1972) and Burstow (1992) outline how psychiatry is often used to deal with "problem" people, such as women who resist female socialization, who have been rejected or abandoned by husbands, or who are poor.

The impact of this positivist scientific normative discourse on the social construction of incest is that I, as an incest survivor, become positioned as "other" to the norm. This label defines my differences, and those in my family, and suggests the skills I need to acquire to become "normal". The complexity of my life as mother, worker, friend, sister, citizen and lover disappears under this one label. Connections between my incest identity and my other identities are not made visible. The complexity of how I live in the world is not discussed.

In the therapeutic framework premised on the scientific conception of normal, I am taught to strengthen personal boundaries destroyed through the abuse, to regain trust, and take responsibility for my actions. While these skills make sense within the framework of therapy, exercising them within the complexity of a world which has little knowledge of, or interest in, survivor "issues" is a different story. My new skills are often resisted. The responses required of me to remain silent and care for others reproduce my past history (Acker & Feuerverger, 1996). The interaction between my past history (partially recovered), my present life, and the contexts in which I live, is the site I want to investigate to further develop understandings about everyday lives of incest survivors.

Creating Meanings

Growing up in a household whose representation to the world differed greatly from its private face led me to develop a sceptical approach to what I was told about the world. As a child, I survived by reading hidden meanings in what was said. Words were not simple expressions of truth; it was vital to read the nuances they contained correctly in different social contexts. I danced to the required social expectations and could sometimes glimpse whether others embraced the dance or shared my alienation. Later, while working with people with disabilities, I used these reading skills to detect the difference between the social rhetoric of rehabilitation and the systemic unemployment and isolation in which they live.

The experience of recovering incest memories eroded what remained of my belief in a unified self living in a universe governed by natural law. Over the years, the power of my mind kept the process of remembering at bay. When I dropped out of the rational verbal stance that defended against memory recall into how I felt in my body, another story of myself quickly began to emerge. Parts of my body that were numb began to feel, unleashing the frozen timeless past, the voices of an abused child. I lived constantly with the terror of a child whose world disintegrated night after night. I carried her to work, to school, and throughout the tasks of mothering, living in a double sense of reality. When I felt angry or sad, it was difficult to sort out what related to the present conditions of my life and what applied to the past. Even when I was clear, I wasn't always sure how to proceed. The reaction of my family of origin to the "news" of my abuse soon taught me to tolerate multiple versions of truth in the same family. Either that or accept the label of "crazy" applied to those who speak unwelcome truth (Chesler, 1972). Remembering challenged the social frameworks through which I had constructed my survival and left me inhabiting a world of partial truths.

A post-structuralist formulation of psychology locates individual formation within social discourses. As Chris Weedon says: "the site of this battle for power is the subjectivity of the individual and it is a battle in which the individual is an active protagonist" (1987:41). Embracing a post-structural view of the self as shifting within social discourses assisted me in hanging onto my own complexity. My conception of myself was not reduced to a singular identity of incest survivor, an "other" I needed to fix in order to gain normalcy. Rather, I maintained some sense of living as a competent adult, as well as a child staring into the face of horror. When I was unable, within most social contexts, to weave these identities together, I became aware of the social regulation which occurs through discursive beliefs and practices.

Through the disruption of unity, of essential categories and binary opposites, and by attending to suppressed tensions, post-structuralists render hidden power relations visible, creating new meanings (Flax, 1990). The purpose of analysis is not to discover the "truth", but to create as many layers of meaning as possible. A post-structural psychology inhabits a world of partial meanings rather than universal truth. What follows is a partial reading of a white, middle-class, able-bodied lesbian incest survivor who used dissociation, strict boundaries between public face and private feelings, and constriction as primary survival tools in a straight and structured world. There are many different incest survivor experiences. My work is a fragment adding to other incest survivors' writing on these issues, in order to enlarge the current mapping of the lives of those who experience incest.

Between 1989 and 1993 I consistently wrote in journals about events which disturbed me. These narratives were driven by parts of me that had lived mostly in silence protected by my public face. Writing has been part of the process through which my places of silence have been brought to speech. Because I have little experience with bringing this voice directly into the work I do, articulating meanings of the stories has been slow, frustrating and terrifying work.

To you, the reader, these stories may feel as if I have dropped my drawers in public. I can picture what my WASP grandmother and mother would say and the stern self-righteousness with which they would say it. Their primary concern would be to protect the family name, to not behave in an "unsuitable" fashion. My response is to ask at what cost to children and women is this protection bought? For me, the price of silence is too high, personally and politically.

Chapter 2

AN OPEN LETTER TO JUDITH LEWIS HERMAN

I *have let go of captivity in bits and pieces, clinging to its familiarity like a child to its mother.*

Having begun to reclaim her forgotten history, the survivor wakes up to a myriad of explanations about how she is to understand her experience and live her life. Like washing on a line, these theories flap in a contradictory wind, creating sound and limited insight constrained by the pegs that hold them.

Dear Judith,

Your book *Trauma and Recovery* has provided a powerful catalyst through which I have been able to articulate my points of connection to and alienation from the therapeutic literature on incest. This letter is intended to explore how the subject "incest survivor" is constituted through your diagnosis of complex post-traumatic stress disorder and more broadly within discourses of medicalization. I'm arguing against the practices of institutionalized diagnosis. My intention is not to contribute to the current backlash against grassroots work with women and children, which is spreading to the mental health professions, but to deepen the moral alliances between survivors and the therapists who support their work.

As a survivor of childhood sexual abuse responding to *Trauma and Recovery*, I am aware that my thoughts may be interpreted as the result of "unfinished" work or representative of the "stage of recovery" I may be in (Greenspan, 1993). Sometimes this thought paralyses me, making it impossible to say anything at all. However, I also believe insights can be gained through reflection from different social locations: you, as a professional creating change within the psychiatric community, me, as an incest survivor reconnecting past, present and future; mind, body and feeling; old patterns and new possibilities.

Complex Post-Traumatic Stress Disorder

As you know, you have developed a new diagnostic category, complex post-traumatic stress disorder, to make sense of the experience and recovery process a survivor of prolonged trauma experiences. In doing so, you separate the experiences of those surviving such trauma as combat, disasters and rape – those who may be diagnosed with post-traumatic stress disorder – from others whose sense of identity, capacity to relate and create meaning is profoundly affected by prolonged traumatic experiences. The impact of these experiences on the survivor's behaviour is outlined in seven categories:

1. A history of subjugation to totalitarian control over a prolonged period (months to years). Examples include hostages, prisoners of war, concentration camp survivors, and survivors of some religious cults . . . survivors of domestic battering, childhood physical or sexual abuse, and organized sexual exploitation.

2. Alterations in affect regulation, including persistent dysphoria, chronic suicidal preoccupation, self-injury, explosive or extremely inhibited anger (may alternate), compulsive or extremely inhibited sexuality (may alternate).

3. Alterations in consciousness, including amnesia or hypermnesia for traumatic events, transient dissociative episodes, depersonalization/derealization, reliving experiences, either in the form of intrusive post-traumatic stress disorder symptoms or in the form of ruminative preoccupation.

4. Alterations in self-perception including a sense of helplessness or paralysis of initiative, shame, guilt, and self-blame, sense of defilement or stigma, sense of complete difference from others (may include sense of specialness, utter aloneness, belief that no person can understand, or nonhuman identity).

5. Alterations in perceptions of the perpetrator, including pre-occupation with relationship with perpetrator (includes pre-occupation with revenge), an unrealistic attribution of total power to perpetrator ... idealization or paradoxical gratitude, a sense of special or supernatural relationship acceptance of belief systems or rationalizations of perpetrator.

6. Alterations in relationships with others, including isolation, withdrawal, disruption in intimate relationships, repeated search for a rescuer (may alternate with isolation and with-drawal), persistent distrust, repeated failures of self-protection.

7. Alterations in systems of meaning, loss of sustaining faith, sense of hopelessness and despair.
   (Herman, 1992: 121)

As you indicate, professionals often do not understand the link between past history and the wide variety of present day symptoms among survivors of childhood sexual abuse. Through an accurate diagnosis, and education about the effects of trauma, as well as detailing key aspects of the recovery process, you hope to change the negative attitudes many professionals hold about survivors of childhood sexual abuse (123).

By drawing parallels between socially legitimated experiences of trauma (hostages, concentration camp survivors) and experiences of abused wives and children, you seek recognition and credibility for the conditions of many women's and children's lives. This framing of my life through the metaphor of captivity is powerful, personally and socially. I recognize more fully how my body, thoughts, actions and beliefs were fashioned by the demands of violence and by life in my family. My survival is remarkable even to me. Your work, and that of other feminists, to create spaces which legitimize my experiences facilitates my willingness to break silence about the conditions of my life.

Insidious Trauma[4]
Paralleling my experience to that of hostages and concentration camp sur-vivors, however, also obscures important differences in survivors' power and privilege which affect the recovery process and political meanings they bring to their experiences. Based on my symptoms, your diagnosis constructs my

present day life as the same as that of a hostage or a concentration camp survivor. In fact, an individual's social location with regard to race, class, gender, sexual orientation and disability, and their access to power and privilege also shapes their experience of trauma (Kadi, 1996). In addition, there are multiple differences in these social and historical events which impact on how individuals understand their experience and rebuild their lives.

For example, questions of responsibility may pose different problems in the everyday lives of hostages, concentration camp survivors and sexual abuse survivors. Your diagnosis of complex post-traumatic stress disorder constitutes survivors as victims of totalitarian control (121). Understanding myself as a victim reduces my self-blame, but it does not assist me in assuming responsibility for my life. The questions I struggle with regarding my responsibility towards aging family members and participation in extended family life will not necessarily be those struggled with by hostages and concentration camp survivors. Because more than my compliant self is present in these struggles over responsibility (or I wouldn't be struggling), they represent crucial opportunities to redefine the landscape of my life. These questions also have the potential to develop critiques of normative social relations which will vary according to the different nature of survivor experiences. By obscuring these differences in your diagnostic category, Judith, possibilities for social change are reduced. The survivor remains focussed on attaining "normal" life and overcoming her pathology.

Depending on their social locations, survivors of prolonged trauma may also experience the impact of "insidious trauma", the daily erosion to "soul and spirit", the constant knowledge of vulnerability to violence, economic hardship or revilement that marginalized groups face (Root, in Brown, 1995:107). My ability to "recover" is affected by the on-going oppression I live as a woman, which echoes my childhood captivity. I am both held in on-going captivity and struggling to break free of it. The barrage of images of women as sexual objects, of glorified male violence in sports and through film, and of the intact nuclear family as the site of care and nurturance, must be negotiated on a daily basis. The media both sensationalizes and trivializes a survivor's experience (Armstrong, 1994). The courts examine women's responsibility for men's actions (Armstrong, 1983; Herman, 1996). Life in the present recalls the violation of the past on a daily basis in ways that are likely very different for a hostage or a concentration camp survivor. News of kidnapping, war, and anti-semitism in the daily media don't have the same traumatic effect on me that they might have on survivors of these specific experiences.

Differences based on race, class and gender positionings may compound or soften the effects of trauma experiences. For example, my race and class privilege allow me to afford safe housing. This protects me from the potential retraumatization of living within an unsafe home environment. Within the general category of survivor there are many different patterns of powerlessness and privilege. These need to be understood within the therapeutic process and used within the process of reclaiming the self (Kadi, 1996). A single diagnosis of complex post-traumatic stress disorder does not capture the nuanced complexity of how trauma lives on in a survivor's everyday life (Rosenberg, 1997).

By separating experiences of prolonged trauma from those of "ordinary" life, important linkages between normative social relations and experiences of violence may also be obscured. Butler (1994) discusses the arbitrary boundary drawn around trauma, separating it from normal life. It is worthwhile to ask: how numb does someone have to be to tolerate working in a fish processing plant or on an assembly line? How dissociated does a person need to be to withstand the privileging of sexes or classes? How much distrust is essential in the daily betrayals of white people towards people of colour? What possibilities exist to disrupt normative social relations if connections are drawn across the prolonged traumas of "everyday" life? You end *Trauma and Recovery,* Judith, with a discussion of the survivor's participation in the "common" and the "ordinary" as signs of recovery. Given the "insidious trauma" which underlies many people's "ordinary" life, I wonder what it is you wish to celebrate in reinforcing "normal" as the goal of recovery.

Similarly, you mention the importance of the survivor's connection to a supportive community in everyday life. Interestingly, the "communities" you discuss – war veterans societies, therapy groups, family and friends – are relatively small, closed communities. The communities the survivor negotiates on a daily basis and where she spends most of her time – at work, in the neighbourhood – are not mentioned in your discussion. For me, even with white middle-class privilege, negotiating these everyday relations remains the most difficult task. They are constantly changing, and public notions of private responsibility for trauma dominate. Your narrow definition of community obscures the survivor's daily struggle to deal with domination while possessing a new awareness of her history and its costs. There is no discussion of how the community could support the survivor by working to end violence against women and children, or to reduce the impact of "insidious trauma".

The concept of insidious trauma (Root, 1992) may also help explain the contradictory nature of your presentation of the recovery process. In *Trauma and Recovery* I'm told my life will settle down and become more ordinary; that I will regain trust in myself as well as in important relationships; that my self-esteem will be repaired; my physical symptoms will be under control; that I will have reconstructed a system of meaning which includes the trauma and will have a narrative of the trauma and can tolerate the feelings associated with it. On the page before, I'm told my symptoms may reappear under stress (203,212,213). On the one hand I recover, on the other hand, I don't.

Realizing the impact insidious trauma has on my attempts to recover assists me in living the contradictory rollercoaster of this process. The therapeutic literature on incest understands the impact of insidious trauma in individual terms: survivors "triggered" by events in the present resembling events in the past (Bass & Davis, 1988). What this individual focus and locus of responsibility misses are the ways in which social relations in the present contain the same power dynamics as those in the past. Seeing how "insidious trauma" erodes my efforts to recover reduces my self blame when my life seems anything but "ordinary".

While therapy teaches the survivor to reconnect body and feeling and to listen to the messages from that reconnection, the general social context will not support the survivor in this work. Brown states that denial and minimalization are necessary to cope with "insidious trauma" (1995). Most women live out degrees of constriction fulfilling their caretaking roles. Given how capitalism severs the public from private, mind from body and feeling, and individual from community, those who consciously attempt to connect body, mind, feeling and spirit are extraordinary, not ordinary. Through the struggle to connect, the survivor engages in politically transformative work which remains unseen and unacknowledged in a diagnostic model that asserts normal life as its goal.

The insidious trauma of daily life rips open my traumatic past, exposing the raw hurt of betrayal and the need to reach towards life from a place of despair. Social denial of insidious trauma, to which you inadvertently contribute, Judith, leaves me alone in negotiating how to connect mind, body, emotions and spirit in an environment designed to separate them. Ironically, if I embrace the normalcy you suggest, then the social visibility of trauma you seek in your work will be reduced (Tal, 1996). I'm surprised that attaining "normal" life becomes your strategy for change, given your eloquent presentation of the captivity in which many women and children live.

Social Regulation Through Discourses of Normativity

By ignoring differences in social power and privilege, medical and scientific diagnostic discourses reinforce normativity. They construct social issues as individual problems and deviations from societal norms. Diagnosis also plays an administrative function, as it is required in institutionalized fee-for-service and delineates the professional boundaries between therapist and client (Greenspan, 1993).

Through creating a new diagnostic category which insightfully describes the abusive power relations in which I grew up, you seek recognition for me as an incest survivor, Judith, based on your professional experience. My symptoms become legitimate through your portrayal of my life as a victim. Because of the social regulation of normativity, individual deviations from "normal" behaviour require explanations from professionals to achieve legitimacy (Foucault in Rabinow, 1984:165). My role within this diagnostic construction of myself is to overcome the symptoms of my victimhood to attain "normal" experience.

If achieving "normal" is the outcome of the therapeutic process and a measure of the way in which an individual contributes to the social good (Venn, 1984), then, in therapeutic terms, I can assess my "progress" based on my ability to sustain relationships, have hope, be physically and emotionally embodied and to reduce my self-blame and dissociative tendencies. The result is that I end up vacillating between a quest for self-perfection (if only I did x then y would not occur) and self-blame at being unable to achieve and maintain normal. This preoccupation with striving to maintain normative standards of behaviour keeps individuals focussed on their individual lives, rather than on social relations in which they live. In this way, attention is diverted from actions potentially directed at social change, to those concerning individual change.

The focus on my pathology within the diagnostic process regulates how I and others understand our experiences of violation and their on-going impact. Parker et al (1995) describe this process as positioning in which "a place is marked out for them and a set of behaviours and experiences is defined for them" (39). The reduction of my experience into the pairing survivor-victim renders invisible skills I have acquired as a competent friend, mother, worker and learner. The places where I have learned trust, to have hope, where I have been physically and emotionally embodied (no matter how minimally) and where I have been able to sustain relationships, disappear under the diagnostic criteria. I am left faced with all I am unable to do, rather than celebrate what I have partially achieved. The process of confronting past trauma requires mobilizing every ounce of desire for life; all the skills that a survivor can find to keep herself alive. Concentrating on what is wrong with me does not affirm the strengths I bring to this work, or my capacity to grow and change. Deepening my acknowledgement of past trauma and its effects in the present requires me to develop a sense of self which knows and trusts my abilities. A diagnosis dissolves my sense of strengths and abilities rather than reinforcing them. Although you seek my empowerment Judith, diagnosing me replays my history and reinforces my sense of powerlessness and lack of worth.

The regulatory power of diagnosis, which creates and is sustained by a dichotomy between "normal" and "other", separates survivors from the experiences of other women. If the effects of my captivity are named on a continuum with other women (Kelly, 1987)[5], then consciousness about the oppression in which all women live is maintained. I am not flipped into a state of "abnormality" that I must "overcome" when I seek help. The assumption you make in proposing a new diagnosis is that some women can handle their oppression, and others, due to its severity, cannot. Women's collective outrage at their captivity, the exile they live from their bodies and from their knowledge, disappears under the therapeutic blanket (Butler, 1992).

Writing in a psychiatric milieu locates your work within medical and scientific practices that carry a regulatory power to draw the boundaries of sanity and insanity, normal and abnormal and construct the patient's role and responsibilities. Foucault (1984) describes the historical evolution of psychiatric practice. Current practice carries many traces of this historical development. While madness had previously been constructed in terms of sin, the growing importance of reason changed how madness was understood. Foucault says:

> The obscure guilt that once linked transgression and unreason is thus shifted; the madman as a human being originally endowed with reason, is no longer guilty of being mad; but the madman, as a madman, must feel morally responsible for everything within him that may disturb morality and society, and must hold no one but himself responsible for the punishment he receives. (145)[6]

The process of treatment systematically observed, judged and condemned those who were mad to create remorse and self-correction. Madness became regarded as a social failure to which genetic weakness and poor environment are linked (Parker et al, 1995). As the source of healing, the doctor represents authority based on order, morality and the family. Increasingly through the work of Freud, the functions of the asylum become embodied in the doctor-patient relationship (Foucault, 1984:163,165). This relationship is character-ized by "moral modes of confession" in which the patient comes to believe the doctor's interpretation in accounting for their distress (Foucault in Parker et al, 1995: 22). Greenspan's critique of psychiatric practice highlights these same historical elements: the emphasis on reason and on the psychic not the social; the view that emotional suffering represents a disease and the power of the fatherly doctor to use his knowledge to provide a cure (1993: xxxi, xxxii).

The feminist critique of psychiatry also unpacks the layers of social power and privilege underlying the historical development of psychiatry. There is a gendered difference in power within this system. Burstow reports that "97% of all psychiatrists are male", while women outnumber men as patients with "mental disorders" by a ratio of 2 to 1 (1992: 33,34).[7]

Normal and abnormal experiences are defined by the life experiences and expectations of white, middle-class, heterosexual, able-bodied men. As Parker et al describe:

> On the one hand the classic female role demands a set of behav-
> iours and experiences which, judged against an ungendered
> norm, are clinically neurotic . . . On the other hand resistance
> against that norm is liable to be interpreted as deviation. (1995: 40)

Within psychiatric practise, problems associated with class and race oppres-sion are also viewed in individualistic terms through the gaze of a white, middle-class, male clinician (Parker et al, 1995: 44-46).

Laura Brown describes the male bias in creating diagnoses in her critique of the *Diagnostic and Statistical Manual of Mental Disorders* (1987) *DSM III-R*. Defining post-traumatic stress disorder, the *DSM III-R* says "the person has experienced an event that is outside the range of human experience" (1995:100), for example, a natural disaster, war, an unpredictable accident. For women, trauma includes unusual events as well as those of everyday life. Although this definition changed in the *DSM-IV,* it seems unlikely that the male gaze underlying the system of diagnosis has altered. As Paula Caplan's discussion of her attempts to intervene in the development of the *DSM-III-R* and the *DSM-IV* demonstrates, psychiatrists continue to minimize interventions by well-qualified professionals who do not support their points of view (1995).

Although, Judith, you critique the arbitrariness of the diagnostic process through your description of psychiatrists wanting to add masochistic personality disorder to the diagnostic manual – "how little rational argument seemed to matter" (117) – by simply proposing a new diagnosis, you continue to support this process. While I believe you are seeking credibility for high numbers of women who have been abused and who are in contact with psychiatry, I question your support of a system which is so fundamentally biased against the realities of women's lives, and does not acknowledge the impact of insidious trauma. Given the regulatory power of psychiatry, however, I understand your efforts to create change from within the system.

But how effective can the change in wording to complex post-traumatic stress disorder be without broader systemic change? To draw from another context, during the twenty years in which I have been involved with people with disabilities, there has been considerable debate about and change in the language through which people are described, from "mentally retarded" to "mentally handicapped" to "developmentally delayed". Some of the change occurs to relieve the stigma of having the condition, but the regulation of creating an "other" to the norm doesn't disappear (Goffman, 1963). The systemic oppression people with disabilities face remains pervasive and invisible, despite a shift in language to create possibilities for people. By moving the labels from "somatization disorder", "borderline personality disorder" and "multiple personality disorder" to "complex post-traumatic stress disorder", you may be riding a similar merry-go-round.

Social Regulation Through Psychiatry

Psychiatry is a system of treatment as well as a practice in which diagnoses are defined. Forms of psychiatric treatment include not only the therapy you mention, Judith, but drugs, electroshock, and committal to an institution. These treatment conditions often replay an individual's experience of captivity and violation. I am surprised you do not explore this within your discussion. Backed by the legal power to incarcerate and to silence individuals through declaring them incompetent, psychiatric treatment carries an enormous regulatory social function, reestablishing physical and emotional control. Seeing my father undergo electroshock "treatment" was a powerful lesson in the violence psychiatry perpetuates.

For many psychiatric survivors, treatment resembles brutality, not help. Kate Millett describes her experience in a psychiatric institution saying:

The bin itself is insane, abnormal, a terrifying captivity, an irrational deprivation of every human need – so that maintaining reason within it is an overwhelming struggle. After a certain time many victims collapse and agree to be crazy, they surrender. (1990: 218)

In their edited collection of psychiatric survivors' experiences Burstow and Weitz (1988) graphically portray violations perpetrated through drugs and electroshock. These captive adult "psychiatric survivors" were subjected to the humiliation of needing permission to go to the bathroom, or not being permitted to wear their own clothes. Chesler outlines how medication and shock treatment have replaced such historical treatments as the strait jacket, solitary confinement, brain surgery and systemic physical violence (1972: 104). In her discussion for feminist therapists working with psychiatric survivors, Burstow (1992) describes in some detail the coercive techniques used by psychiatric professionals when patients cease taking their medication, and the discrimination psychiatric survivors face within the medical profession as a whole.

Burstow outlines how medication – neuroleptics in particular, which are most commonly prescribed – can block the production of dopamine in the body, which "affects feeling, impedes perception, movement control and affect" (1992:30). Capponi (1992), in her personal account of life as a psychiatric survivor, refers to the grey fog of life on medication.

How can someone begin to sort through the process of remembering their past and reclaiming their history when their feelings and perceptions are already altered?[28] How will they know what is real for them? Taking prescription medication would teach me that living in my body and reclaiming my memories was too impossible a task to be undertaken. Within this kind of treatment regime, people learn to obey, to "act normal" if it prevents further violations. This continues captivity and prevents them from reclaiming different parts of their experience. Your efforts to advocate within a system which demonstrates such a violent and coercive agenda deeply troubles me.

Feminist Therapy
Because discourses of normativity carry such regulatory power, you are not the only feminist therapist, Judith, to construct your work within its frameworks. At this point I'll turn from directly discussing your book *Trauma and Recovery* to examining how discourses of normativity are played out in other writing about incest survivors.

Feminist therapy seeks to provide an alternative to psychiatric treatment by reestablishing the links between individual experience and social systems of power and privilege, and by positioning the therapist as supporting rather than directing the client's therapeutic process (Greenspan, 1993). However, discourses of normativity continue to permeate feminist therapeutic practice. Burstow points out that feminist efforts to reframe women's experience have not been consistent. Feminist therapists may not be sufficiently critical of psychiatry, resulting in their participation in committing their clients to institutions and their unwillingness to work with psychiatric survivors. Some may continue to use psychiatrically-defined diagnoses such as "multiple personality disorder". Differences of opinion among feminist therapists over suicide illustrate this difficulty. While some therapists believe empowerment includes the client's right to kill herself (Burstow, 1992), others, like you, would commit a client to ensure her safety (Herman, 1992). Similarly, the constant admonishment to resist pathologizing women's coping mechanisms – dissociation, splitting, and cutting – in much of the writing by feminist therapists speaks to psychiatry's power to define and regulate discourses of normativity (Burstow, 1992; Butler, 1992). While you share a desire to advocate on women's behalf with other feminist therapists, Judith, on-going critical analysis is required to identify the underlying patterns of pathology and social control which maintain women's subjugation.

Self-help

Feminists have also used the low cost availability and popularity of self-help to try and increase ways of helping women (Burstow, 1992; Tal, 1996). Some feminist therapists articulate self-help's role in establishing basic safety routines (Burstow, 1992; Butler, 1992). However, the underlying discourses within self-help reinforce normative agendas, highlighting the individual over the systemic and focussing on returning to "normal".

The world view of self-help is one in which pain is "dysfunctional" and individuals are the cause of their problems (Butler, 1992). The impact of insidious trauma on incest survivors' lives remains invisible. When I read *The Courage to Heal,* the well-known self-help handbook for women survivors of childhood sexual abuse, I am left feeling exhausted and guilty for all the actions I am not taking on my own behalf, for all the patterns I am unable to alter. With its clear message that I can be a "survivor" who overcomes the effects of my violation, I can only be perceived as perpetuating my victimhood, my pathology, when I am unable or unwilling to act on my own behalf.

In this perspective lies a refusal to acknowledge the on-going depth and persistence of the effects of childhood sexual abuse. It encourages me, once again, to suppress the pain. In moments when I can help myself, I know what to do. But moments when I can do nothing but bear the pain of my existence in the depth of my trauma are not the times to tell me what I could be doing to help myself. In fact, this encourages me to distract myself through action, rather than move through the pain by allowing it to surface and be experienced. Although one of the intentions of *The Courage To Heal* is to communicate that I am not the only person who has gone through this experience and thereby encourage me, its overall impact is discouragement and alienation. I have wondered if its intended but unacknowledged audience is primarily women whose lives depend on not re-entering a psychiatric institution.

This creation of a feminist survivor identity continues the fragmentation I created as a child in order to survive. The same coupling between survivor/victim which limits the acknowledgement of my strengths in your work, Judith, is present here. On the one hand I was a victim in the past and what happened wasn't my fault. On the other hand, I am now expected to behave as a survivor, not as a victim. The word "survivor" resonates closest to the mask with which I greet the world. She's the one who figured out how to survive, how to "fit in" and "look good". Now she's supposed to manage the symptoms of my trauma history. This survivor identity is not constructed to accept the pain resulting from the past, nor to integrate it into my sense of self. In fact I am a survivor, I am vulnerable to being revictimized and I am more than either of these two things. What I long for is to affirm and relax into the complexity of my being, which will both include and transcend my experiences of childhood sexual abuse. As long as I remain within the survivor/victim pairing, this integration will not take place. In their desire to belong to the women's community and to cope with their lives, women may become good feminist clients within this discourse and continue to deny and minimize their pain.

Within mainstream self-help groups such as Alcoholics Anonymous, co-dependency and twelve-step programs, the lack of analysis of women's oppression, the shallowness of the approach and the subjugation to a higher power are seen as problematic for women (Burstow, 1992; Greenspan, 1993; Butler, 1992). The psychiatric dictate that the problem is all in your head is now changed to it's all in your family (Greenspan, 1993). The conditions of captivity are recreated through obedience to the self-help groups' prescriptions for living. They remind me of the rules I constructed as a child to maintain a sense of safety, and the symbolic gestures through which I kept a spark of hope alive. These rules are constructed to cope with, rather than experience, the depth of underlying pain.

Feminist self-help groups are designed to increase self-knowledge and problem-solving in an environment of mutual support (Wycoff, 1980; Ernst & Goodison, 1985). In Wycoff's early work on women helping themselves she says, "after I made the decision to take responsibility for my life and really live it, I also made a decision to love and nurture myself" (1980: 157). That decision in my life is made in fits and starts over years of work, not through a time-limited group experience. It requires feeling enough sustained trust and affection within the therapeutic relationship to allow me to summon the energy to do more than just survive. The encouragement to "take charge" of my life inhibits the exploration of the depth of pain and damage left from the violation and contributes to my alienation from some feminist writing.

There is potential within self-help groups for relationships with people who may understand. This links back, Judith, to the examples of community you mention as places where survivors can establish some connection. Sufficient depth and containment may not be present in these relationships, however, to create the necessary internal shifts within an individual required to feel understood. Indeed, with the complexity of individual histories and coping styles present in any self-help group, these may be more suited to enhancing self-awareness than to developing long-term, stable, trusted relationships. Belonging may come to depend on maintaining the group narrative about their experiences rather than on changing their lives.

What I find most alienating in the feminist self-help literature, and most destructive of building community and a strong political voice, is the assertion of the possibility of healing, recovery. While I have "recovered" in the sense of regaining more of my past, a greater sense of life, more experience of bodily sensation and emotion, and being less driven by the dictates of past captivity, I would not describe this process as healing with its definitional overlay of a cure or as a return to normal (Herman, 1992). Incest shattered my sense of self, my capacity to relate to others, and my ability to act from a place of desire rather than survival. It is from acknowledging the depth and irreparable nature of the damage that a survivor's politics are born. The violation of one more child becomes unacceptable when the costs are clearly articulated and visible. The hope that can be found must grow from the ruins of a shattered life, not from denial of the costs or false promises of restoration. The promise of healing within self-help becomes the containment of political action within a discourse of normativity focussed on the individual achievement of "normal".

Survivor Accounts

Like self-help, survivor accounts have developed predominantly through a therapeutic lens[9]. Describing this result of early feminist work aimed at creating visibility and social change, Armstrong says "it was not our intention merely to start a long conversation" (1994:7). As you know through your work Judith, the alternate discourses provided by feminist theories, combined with/supported by underlying sense of a women's community, created the amount of social recognition that exists (Tal, 1996). However, in describing the inherent disruption of survivor speech by dominant social discourses, Alcoff & Gray conclude that "the tendency, however, will always be for the dominant discourse to silence such speech or, failing this, to channel it into non-threatening outlets" (1993: 268). Accounts which encourage sensationalism and voyeurism or mediation by an "expert" tend to marginalize survivor speech (Williamson, 1994; Tal, 1996; Alcoff & Gray, 1993). Mainstream publishing plays a dominant role in framing the type of survivor experience which receives public attention (Tal, 1996).

Through these dynamics of power within social discourses, published survivor accounts focus predominantly on portraying the experience of incest while growing up and on the process of recovery. They demonstrate the creativity through which children construct their survival (Miller, 1990). Some are fictional representations (Fraser, 1988; Gahlinger,1993; MacDonald, 1996) while others are autobiographical (Wisechild, 1988; Danica, 1988). All of them are difficult to read, many are moving, some bring me insight, others resonate with aspects of my history. Different accounts have resonated at different times in my process. Some, such as Randall's (1987) use of photographs of her abuser, have pushed the edges of my silence into speech.

In recreating a world of memory and therapeutic recovery (Alcoff & Gray, 1993), many survivor accounts provide the client's perspective on your work, Judith.[10] In addition, the linearity of storytelling – with a beginning, middle and end – leaves an impression that the process of therapy and remembering results in a life that is better, rather than one that is simply different (Hoppen, 1994).

The questions I am asking about connections between normative discourses, as I experience them at work, in relationships, and with family remain unaddressed in your work. What I need to hear are not the ways in which I can "heal" or "recover", but what it is like for women who have been in this process longer than I have. How has their relationship to incest changed? What happens as they move through their life span? What have they learned that might be useful to me? How is it different for women who are not living with the race and class privilege of my own? Having landed in a therapeutic box, how do survivors collectively work for social change?

Stories of silence and disenfranchisement located in different race and class positionings than my own often spark my creativity and my desire to break through my oppression (Walkerdine & Lucey, 1989; Pratt, 1991, 1984; Lorde, 1984; Walker, 1982). From my perspective, the beginning point for further survivor accounts is to resist normative therapeutic frameworks which focus on recovery and to connect our experience as survivors to the regulatory power of discourses of normativity.

Survivor Differences, Survivor Gifts

Through your yardstick of normal, Judith, my development is seen in abnormal terms. If the requirement that my behaviour be measured according to socially established norms is abandoned, it becomes possible to generate a different understanding of the therapeutic process, as well as survivor experiences. Some feminist therapists have reframed normativity through acknowledging insidious trauma in their practice (Burstow, 1992; Butler, 1992; Brown, 1995). In this model, pain is a "normal" part of women's experience. Their emphasis is on helping women carry their history and knowledge of on-going subjugation (which varies according to race and class positionings), as well as their consciousness, and still connect with the power of life. Laura Brown points toward the transformative potential of therapy when she says:

> How . . . can we help them to reconstruct their world views with the knowledge that evil can and does happen? . . . How can we facilitate their integration of their painful new knowledge into an ethic of compassion, feeling with, struggling with the web of life with which they relate? (1995: 109, 110)

Burstow outlines the importance of authenticity "when we realise our connectedness with all that exists", and of power – the capacity "to realize projects . . . to define/change the world" (1992: 2). These feminist therapists speak of help, not of healing. Their models offer potential to link therapeutic process with the social discourses in and through which survivors live.

Rather than focusing on returning to "normal", these theorists connect an individual woman's experience to on-going conditions of oppression. Because of the entrenchment of social discourses based on individualized pathology, sustained critical consciousness by the therapist, and by those individuals and theoretical and practical frameworks that support her work, is necessary.

Changing assumptions based on normativity also allows for a reconception of the therapeutic process. Although, Judith, you conceptualize the recovery process as a linear progression through stages, you also sometimes describe it as a spiral. For me, the most difficult memories, the deepest grief and greatest struggle to connect into the world in an embodied way come as I grow stronger and can tolerate and encompass more of my experience both in the past and the present. My engagement with my history will not just reoccur as I move through the stages of my life, but as it becomes part of my forma- tion, so too will it become part of my growth. I will continue to spiral down through the horror in order to reclaim my life. My capacity to engage in the horror, both past and present, has strengthened. Further work is required to fully articulate the implications of a model of spiralling recovery.

When children who grow up in captivity are seen through the lens of normativity, their development and the survival skills they have learned are seen as being abnormal. If this mold is broken Judith, what potential strengths can be identified and developed in these skills? Survivors develop powerful skills of observation, listening and attunement (Miller, 1981). These can take them out of their bodies and away from focussing on their own desires, feelings, sensations. These skills are often presented as "problems" to be overcome. But they are also highly developed abilities. My question is how to learn to use these abilities without being taken away from myself.

Similarly, the double-think with which a survivor lives (Herman,1992), between how I am expected to act to survive and how am I feeling, has the potential (shared by people living other forms of marginalization) to develop a critical analysis between how I am told society operates and what I experience (Narayan, 1989). While therapists talk of naming the oppression women live as part of a therapeutic process which would help to develop the intuitive critical analysis of double-think, I find no further mention made in the therapeutic literature on incest of ways to help this capacity grow (Brown, 1995; Burstow, 1992; and Butler, 1992).

Once I have become more aware and accepting of the splits within my selves which helped me survive, there is enjoyment as well as pain, in living such complex and contradictory richness. My creativity has formed and continues to inform who I am. While often frustrating, I live with the daily knowledge of the powerful potential within the self to create and sustain life. The extraordinary courage, endurance and strength of survivors to become fully alive, in spite of the costs, has the potential to challenge social norms which deaden sensation, emotion and spirit. While my work begins to develop this understanding, more work from survivors located differently in terms of race and class positionings would further layer this knowledge.

Beyond the acknowledgement of survivor gifts as a counterpoint to normative conceptions of survivor experience, a different theory of survivor development has the potential to generate new insights. Sandra Butler comments on the fundamental altering violation creates when she says:

> Once a woman has faced the malevolence of someone she
> trusts, admires or loves, someone she expects to hold her interests
> in at least as equal importance to her own, she is forever altered.
> Such violations change who she would have become and how
> she lives the rest of her life. (1994: audiotape)

As someone who dissociated from the time I was a young child, in order to survive, dissociation has fundamentally shaped my formation as a person. The subtleties underlying this formation can be lost in a theory which only sees my pathology. Terr outlines how dissociation begins with self-hypnosis (1994: 87). Culbertson highlights how the extremity of the survivor's experience shares similarities to the experience of mystics in awareness of other levels of reality. She says:

> The survivor experience is in important ways then a mystical
> one, in that it involves states of consciousness, reported experiences,
> and visions reported by mystics . . . Transcendent experiences by
> mystics . . . Transcendent experiences . . . may seem forgotten
> because unsaid, though the survivor lives with a sense of home-
> sickness for an experience, even a place (as mystics and shamans
> often report on a 'geography' of the metaphysical) that cannot
> be otherwise explained. The survivor reports a sense of depression
> and confusion that is perhaps the suppressed experience of this
> other reality, this suppression of a desire to reenter in the body
> what is, whatever else one may call it, clearly another state of
> consciousness. In short, survivors are unwilling, uninitiated,
> unprepared, unschooled mystics. (1995:177)

Drawing parallels between mystical experiences and those of near-death, Walsh (1990) and Fenwick & Fenwick (1995) highlight how this experience is profoundly life changing. According to Walsh, spontaneous mystical journeys are out-of-body experiences with a sense of travel, of meeting spirits and of gaining valuable information. Survivors emerge from near death experiences – in which they have been out of their body – and, in many cases, travel towards a light, with reduced fear of death, an increased belief in the afterlife, more interest in knowledge and learning, more emphasis on caring and helping others than on materialistic goals, more awareness of the preciousness of life, love and relationships (Walsh, 1990:150). Fenwick & Fenwick describe feelings of joy or calm accompanying these experiences, as well as a sense of emotional detachment from the world.

Reading this material, which draws parallels between dissociation and mystical transcendent experiences, I am struck by my unnamed resistance to seeing dissociation in the negative terms employed within the therapeutic literature on incest. Until now, I have had neither the language nor the knowledge to express my grief at the need to return to a pedestrian body after being able to fly. I greet this with as much enthusiasm as Peter Pan being asked to grow up. I am homesick for an experience I cannot even name. I live with a sense of having voyaged, a sense of living with knowledge and connection that cannot be expressed in language, and which, to my puzzlement, others do not seem to share.

While my knowledge of this field is limited, what I want to highlight is my reluctance to give up the pleasures of dissociation and the formative developmental split between my dissociation, on the one hand, and daily life as a silent disciplined captive, on the other. I am left frustrated by the limitations of my abilities to articulate and to act on what I know intuitively. I despair at the length of time things take, the imperfection of the result, and feel lonely because others do not appear to live in the world in the same way. In very concrete ways, I have little experience of acting to achieve my desires unless they are connected to my survival. Realizing my projects within the world requires practice connecting my body, feelings and thoughts in action (Burstow, 1992).

My decision to live in the world rather than in a dissociated place came slowly, over years of work building a relationship with my therapist, in which I knew for certain she wanted to come close to my experiences of the past. The parts of me immersed in the past did not know she was separate from me and needed me to verbalize what I experienced in order to understand and connect to my world, needed language to act as a bridge between us. Staying anchored in the world requires a relationship with myself and a few trusted others with whom I feel alive and taken seriously. The nuances within my experiences of dissociation strongly suggest a need for further theoretical work to understand both its meaning in survivor's lives, as well as its connection to states of altered consciousness.

In articulating the need for further theoretical work, Judith, I am ending where you began. Your work provides a powerful illustration of how assumptions within discourses of normativity remain embedded in efforts to create greater understanding of the impact of violence on adult survivors and children. My experience as an incest survivor will only be understood when the regulatory power of these discourses is challenged. The focus on alleviating individual symptoms must be resisted in order to explore the impact of insidious trauma, the development of survivor strengths and strong political survivor voices, and how daily life can be lived within and beside traumatic experience.

I thank you for all the ways in which your work has both illuminated my life and challenged me towards greater articulation of my experience. In your on-going advocacy on behalf of women, I wish you well.

Sincerely,

Tanya Lewis

Chapter 3

AMPUTATED AFFECTIONS

A family without secrets is rare indeed.
ANNETTE KUHN,
Family Secrets, Acts of Memory and Imagination

Memory becomes a jumble of family photographs and traditions, of laughter, horror, betrayal and confusion. Silence is a habit, a veneer of cooperation and connection.

Michel Foucault introduced the concept of discipline as a form of social power which regulates everyday life by working on and through the body, and operates by establishing minimum standards for individual performance. Performance must meet the minimum standard or face social sanctions, which typically delineate moral and immoral behaviour (in Rabinow, 1984). The standard underlying acceptable family life is that of heterosexual monogamy. Although the father is regarded historically as the head of the family, the role of the mother to ensure "appropriate" care became increasingly important through the nineteenth and twentieth centuries (Donzelot, 1980).

The state plays a role in defining the nature of the family through its legislative power to sanction violations of minimum standards of care, and to encourage the reproduction of certain forms of family life through social assistance (Donzelot, 1980). Policies and procedures attached to social assistance define and regulate what is acceptable and unacceptable within families (Little, 1994). Philanthropy plays a major part in helping to develop effective social assistance interventions (Donzelot, 1980). Underlying state interest is the control and reproduction of the labour force. Therefore, its interventions are aimed predominantly at the working class.

Foucault traces the historical paths of contemporary social discourses which outline the family's responsibility for the health of its members, particularly its children. Aspects of the family's health responsibilities include not only physical care and emotional support and nurturing for its members (Kuhn, 1995), but also the moral development of children (Adams, 1994)[11]. Support for the expectations of other social institutions, such as schools, also becomes part of the family's responsibilities. Social power and privilege are interwoven with these social standards, resulting in a picture of healthy family life that reflects white, middle-class heterosexual values. Idealized images – such as Christmas television specials that portray mom, dad, the children, loving extended family members celebrating in an affluent home – encapsulate this portrait of "health".

Within the standards of care expected of families – to maintain a clean, nurturing, disciplined and moral environment – there is a range of acceptable behaviour. Those who do not meet acceptable standards jeopardize their social "respectability" and are disciplined through public scrutiny of their capacity to meet their responsibilities. In Canada, this is most often done through child welfare agencies, schools, health, or other social workers.

As a child growing up, the maintenance of my family's respectability was an important aspect of family life. My heightened awareness of the importance of respectability probably resulted from my family's lower middle-class economic vulnerability, their middle-class aspirations, as well as their secret of incest. The work of performing myself as a "normal" person, as a member of a "normal" family, was as formative to who I have become as the experience of incest. Behaving "normally" helped me develop key survival skills which assisted me in obtaining an education, in finding and keeping employment, in developing relationships, in maintaining my health and home, as well as caring for my children. My ability to meet social standards upheld my sense of self as someone who was "normal". At the same time, the normative appearance of my family of origin (to those inside as well as outside my family) contributed to my silence, my obedience and my alienation. Little has been written about the impact of normativity on incest survivors' coping strategies or on their silence, lack of trust and alienation. Instead, incest is regarded as an anomaly within the "normal" and "healthy" family portrait, in spite of the acknowledgement of male violence within families (Herman, 1992) including those regarded as socially respectable (Renvoize, 1993). Abuse clearly violates idealized physical boundaries, and emotional and moral responsibilities expected of male family members. The standard of "normal" family life is, however, held in place by medical and social science discourses that position families in which incest occurs as "abnormal", as "other".

In her excellent review of the literature on violence within families,

Faith Elliot summarizes social science explanations of factors contributing to male-perpetrated incest within families, factors that are to explain this "abnormality" (1996). Psychological interpretations are characterized by their focus on the internal pathology of the perpetrators, the mothers, and in some instances, the victims (Steed, 1994; Herman, 1993; Meiselman, 1978). Examples of these representations include mothers who are unable to build solid relationships with their husbands or who are physically absent; fathers who are dominating within their families and passive when confronted by external social authority; daughters who are "seductive" and who have emotional needs that have not been met in appropriate ways.

Another version of this theme portrays the family system as dysfunctional in meeting its members' needs, usually through failure to conform to gender roles (Forward & Buck, 1988). Relationships between husband and wife, between parents and children, or among siblings, are implicated as the "cause" of abuse. Elliot summarizes this perspective, which pervades media, social service and therapeutic approaches to sexual abuse, saying "violence and sexual abuse are constructed as psychological diseases" (1996: 170). In particular, she notes the broader social context impacting on the family. Examples of factors that compound a family's isolation and lack of support include poverty, poor housing and poor social support through neighbours and schools. Structural explanations include the cultural condoning of violence, conflict and stress created by family life, and victimization arising from inequities between men, women and children.

Within the social science disciplines, feminist writers highlight the importance of male power in understanding sexual abuse and of the cultural linkages between violence, sexuality and social constructions of masculinity. Responsibility for regulating men's sexuality and protecting children falls to women. Social work and legal institutions emphasize individual pathology, and fail to impose strong legal sanctions except in cases of the most blatant abuse. As I read this material, many of the factors theorized as contributing to sexual abuse can be seen within my family, including my mother's on-going struggle with a fibrillating heart condition which limited what she could do, her inability to economically support her children, her passivity regarding the conditions of her life, my father's dominance, his self-absorption and his drinking. What strikes me as missing in this construction of my family as "other" is their respectability, all the daily ways they worked to uphold social norms of a family's responsibilities. Here I would include both how we lived as a lower middle-class family, and the healthy values passed on through family life. Our resemblances to other respectable families was greater than our differences. And yet, there was on-going horror.

When I think about my family or have contact with them now, it is as if the scab on a wound is ripped open. Avoidance often seems like the only reliable way to cope. The wound partly results from their continued denial of our shared history, which betrays the values they say they uphold. The wound is also reopened through past lessons learned in my family – focus on the needs of others, be compliant and quiet – which continue in the present. I am left feeling distrustful, fearful, sad, angry and disappointed in my relationships with them. My existence is defined by them now as a member of a clan with a shared history and a sense of obligation to one another. Their sense of family is reinforced by social norms, leaving me with only therapeutic support (which marginalizes my life as "other") to uphold my shattering of their silence. My life as a person with goals, thoughts and needs that are different from theirs are mostly ignored, rendering any sense of my individuality invisible.

At the same time, I know I have been deeply formed by my family's love of beauty in nature, music and literature, their desire for fun, their teaching about living decently and by their emphasis on helping others through action. In embracing these values, I maintain a fundamental tie of loyalty and connection to my family. And I live my relationships with them caught somewhere between avoidance, camaraderie, compassion and grief.

The impact of normativity occurs in the crazy-making (in)congruences between social norms of family and a survivor's experience of family life. In exploring my contradictory experiences within my family through narratives, a more complex picture of a family in which incest occurs emerges: where family is both a site of teaching values and acceptable, healthy behaviour, as well as of profound disrespect for the well-being of its children.

The House

It is such an ordinary house, now that other people live there, that I am surprised when I pass it. As a child, I never crossed its threshold without touching the verandah post: a talisman. I needed its protection for the complicated negotiation required by life in that house. The interior was as claustrophobic as its atmosphere. Care had to be taken to avoid footstools and chairs, hard wooden edges and slippery floors. Photographs, dustables, plants and crocheted doilies cluttered the surfaces. Unspoken nuances, like careful movements, were key to survival in that house.

Family

My aunt, uncle and cousin lived up the street, and another two aunties around the corner. Their presence recreated life in the small Welsh village where they had been born, and the small Canadian village where they grew up. They were short, talkative and energetic, assuming that as family they were always welcome. My mother resented the intrusion of her husband's family into her daily routine; a frosty politeness communicated her displeasure. I found it hard when they came to our house. I was caught in a swirl of emotion and past events I could feel but did not understand. I came to adopt my mother's reserve as my own. We were not to talk about family affairs outside the house. I became uncertain in conversations with my chatty relatives.

My aunties had odd names. Soft Welsh names shortened to fit Anglo-Saxon Canada. I loved the warmth of one aunty's kitchen, the smell of her recent baking and her affection and interest. Another aunty told stories of Wales that taught me to imagine, to long and to dream. A third aunty felt as familiar as a favourite sweater: quiet, warm, accepting.

When I see my father's family now, mostly at funerals, I am surprised by their appearance of respectability. People who work hard, marry, raise their kids, have a little fun along the way. Women who wear skirts and dresses, who drink little and are always nice. Men who drink quite a bit, enjoy playing games and look vaguely hurt and disappointed. Some of them appear to be drifting serenely into old age. They do not seem to have my demons: my father's drive or my mother's reverence for knowledge.

I wonder what they thought of my parents, if they knew of the abuse, the tyranny lived at our house. By their lack of questions about my "odd" behaviour over the last number of years, I doubt they want to know. In moments of sorrow and rage I hold them accountable for their blindness and denial. Despite all the affection they may have had, may still have for me, these are not folks I can count on.

Except for my grandmother, who was fetched faithfully each Sunday by my father for roast beef and television, we saw little of my mother's family. One of her brothers drank, the other brother lived with my grandmother and was "odd". My mother was proud of her United Empire Loyalist background. Although thrift dominated my mother's life even in my day, she had come from a family that was solidly middle-class. She took ballet lessons as a girl. Like many girls at the time, my mother left school after grade eight. It was my mother, not her brother, who should have been encouraged to attend university. As a young woman she had loved the activity, the fun in my father's family. Her middle-class roots married my father's working-class ambition.

As a child, I loved my grandmother's strength, the way she would laugh as we hauled her out of her chair, her knees having given way. My mother resented my grandmother's competence, the ways she had felt pushed aside as a child as not capable. Later, when in her nineties, my grandmother moved to a nursing home, I did not visit very often, siding with my mother against my oldest sister's desire for me to involve myself with her and my grandmother. Something in the relationship between my mother, her mother and my oldest sister warned me of danger, of forbidden territory. Forced in silence to choose, I amputated my affections to survive. Fidelity and love were never simple in that house.

Born the youngest of five children when my parents were in their mid-forties, I grew up with a sense that I had missed all the good parts of my family's life together. They spoke of the old days of living on "the island" most of the year, of cottages rented and people they no longer saw, of the time when "everyone" but my mother sang in my father's church choir. In another way I don't regret having missed those days at all. My parents mellowed as they grew older. I missed the worst of their tyranny and the days of greatest financial hardship.

There were two sets of girls, with my brother stuck in the middle, attempting to bridge the twenty-three year gap between oldest and youngest. Each of the older girls in the pair were seen by my mother as similar, outgoing, vivacious. The second sister was the quiet one buried in a book. We seem dissimilar now, out from under the dictates of family legend. Yet we must have been formed by it as well, because this shadow-sister seems to live a rhythm similar to my own, content with quiet walks or the solitary pleasures of a book. This shadow-sister is not a visceral part of my childhood, although I recall an inexplicable grief when I was five, which could have coincided with her escape to my oldest sister in Montreal.

The sister I grew up with was four years older, wandered, and usually got lost on family vacations. My success at school and her early pregnancies divided our lives into different social experiences, different struggles. As adults we share moments of a sisterhood, a conspiracy so powerful I could fly in our laughter. However, our griefs and struggles are only alluded to, never fully shared. Admitting my vulnerability risks possible judgement or a loss of independence. My mother said we were close, that we played by the hour as children. My memory is ambivalent, as if our loyalties were forged by the needs of family and not by our relationship.

My brother brought the world in through the door when he came with talk of the Cuban missile crisis, of life at the university. He was the son and heir, the focus of attention and scrutiny by my father. From the night I sang too loudly in the bathroom as he struggled to study for his exams, I feared angering him. I was eleven when he married and left home. I cried, wanting to go with him. When I was married, we shared a pleasant connection. I would have said we were close. But as soon as I expressed what lay behind my exterior mask, he was gone.

My oldest sister often returned for holidays, or later, when my mother was ill. She usually carried herself as if she was ready to walk out on stage: made-up, poised, certain not to miss her cue. I liked the excitement of her coming, the trip to Union Station to meet her train. She paid me to wrap her Christmas presents, she took me bird-watching and would sometimes buy a longed-for gift. She is now ill and a sense of duty leads me to question what I owe to her. I can't hold myself in the face of the rage in her eyes, her insistence on maintaining myths that are her truths, and her physical collapse into grief. She wants from me her due as a family member. There will be no acknowledgement of my father's violence or my struggles to live now. Each time I ask myself if I should visit her, my terror keeps me away.

This sister lives in my dreams as dread, the family secrets carved throughout her life in ways I still do not understand. I knew to follow her lead, to keep within the lines she drew. Her rage was silent and dangerous. My mother disliked the way details trailed after her, the make-up left in the bathroom, an unpopular cat that needed a home. My sister helped others and had little time for the drudgery that was my mother's day.

That house had skeletons jangling in the closets with unspoken secrets, hidden anger and grief. When we grew up my siblings and I would sit, during visits together, trying to unravel the stories, learn the secrets. As I regained memories, I grew tired and upset by these efforts, my pain flooding through the numbness of the years.

> *They come at night when I am in bed. A huge shadow, hands groping, invading. I struggle in horror. I am too small. I have not yet learned to get away, to pass out or float away. I shatter into a thousand pieces. Next morning my body wakes and carries on, not knowing I have died. I carry on for years not knowing it was safer now, I could live.*

The drama was off stage, the terror and horror of bedtime forgotten in the numbness of my mother's routine of clean clothes, tidy rooms, three meals

41

a day. I held onto her life raft. I grew enfeebled by her on-going preoccupation with the workings of my body. Maybe this was her way of simultaneously knowing and not knowing, or perhaps she still lived in the years of childhood deaths before penicillin.

In that house of skeletons, that silent battleground, I took my mother's side against my father. I mostly became her daughter, physically timid, intellectual, seeking routine and duty over my father's charisma. Unable and perhaps unwilling to protect me, my mother chose my father over me, loyal to her marriage vow.

My mother was as yielding as a boulder of granite: hard, silent, wounded to the core. She was a person of stifled longings, simple pleasures and uncompromising endurance to her duty. I find it difficult to focus my memory on her, the lens remains diffuse. I think of her often. As I enter mid-life and wear glasses, I see once again her bird-like movements as she played the piano wearing bifocals. Perhaps it is easier to hold onto some connection rather than to know how distant and unseeing she was[12]. Her lessons live on through me as I recycle and compost, and in my horror of wasted food, or of too generous a hand in the stew pot or with toilet paper. I embrace her thrift and resist her sense of duty and decorum that chained her to her family in domestic drudgery and silence. When I was home with young children, I feared the depression of her days, I learned how small her world was.

She was beautiful in a tailored ladylike fashion. We were taught to be neat and tidy, what our good features were. My oldest sister's primping and make-up were frowned on. "To thine own self be true" was the motto my mother taught me and perhaps came to regret.

I am tiny lying in a crib in the alcove of my parents' bedroom. I wake up terrified. Someone is watching me. It is my mother looking angry. I go back to sleep unable to tolerate her face.

What did she find? Was it my mother, my oldest sister, my aunts who checked on me to find the sperm covered face, the sticky necked sleepers of a baby taught to suck her father's penis, choking, inhaling the thick hot liquid? Could they have pretended it was milk? My father would not have cleaned me up.

That became my story with my mother. She acted as the clean up crew. By her rage I learned it was my fault, I was bad. I tried to atone by taking care of her. At least she was predictable, unlike my father.

Later when she was in the hospital with a fibrillating heart unable to contain its pain, I missed the safety of the routines she established, whatever control she was able to exert over them.

Why did she stay? Why didn't my father's family help her? I know the feminist answers to that question[13]. They are not enough.

My father was a bustling charismatic man who sucked attention from the air and lived a public face. He had a cruel angry edge, blind to the needs of those near him. He talked constantly, reassuring himself of his worth, of his existence. He sold custom-tailored clothes and was rarely home, living in a swirl of meetings and work. Flowers grew brilliantly from his sweat. My family sang in four part harmony effortlessly, obedient to his hands' command. I stumbled among them in an uncertain alto, a voice made for the tenor parts reserved for the boys. It is only in his death that I can bear the choral music he loved, longing now, in greater safety, for that soaring connection to him.

My desire to hang out in factories, garages and in working-class pubs comes from him. In his service to the wealthy, he developed an intuitive class analysis which he passed on, along with his blatant anti-semitism and racism.

Bum fucked, mouth fucked, cunt fucked. What difference does it make? I am a garbage pail for my father and his friends. I lie numbed, bruised, cowed, bum in the air. It no longer hurts. I am no longer human.

As I sit here now and recall the flavours and sounds of that childhood, what I remember most powerfully is the tension, the need to watch, modulate and step carefully through the boring routine. The house was most at peace when my parents were at rest, reading or watching TV.

The out of doors acted as a family safety valve for the oppressive tension. Each year we spent a month on a lake near Parry Sound. My brother had a summer bread route by then, to earn money for his next year at university. He would drop by for a visit, lunch and a swim. A family friend arrived every Friday night at dark, bringing barbecued chicken. The abuse didn't stop at the cottage. When I returned there recently, I realised how well I could remember the shape of the land, the curve of the lake as if I had rested connected to the pine trees, the rocks and the water. Oddly enough, it is the noise and confusion of my family that I miss, when everyone would come home or visit the cottage. The chatter of many voices, the laughter and the bustle of activity, the music and the games that drowned out my mother's depression, my parents' sniping at one another. I could relax and enjoy the fun, watchful of too much attention, possible humiliation. Although I was "one of the gang", my struggles went unseen, unacknowledged.

Family games, music and time spent "up north" bond me to my family. When I watched my parents delight in their toddling grandchildren, I could remember their same delight with me, the same games being played that had been played with me, a family living out its pleasure in the promise of another young life. It is these moments, this strong sense of connection through shared activities, as well as all the daily ways my family did what other families do, that make the violence so difficult to assimilate as part of the story. No one, outside of, or within the family circle, penetrated the normative veil of clean clothes, regular meals, or obedient polite children.

School

As a child beginning to go to school, the world was a scary place. Each day I ran past the house with the large barking dog. My mother was furious when I accepted a ride from a stranger. He rescued me from my anxiety, waiting for my sister when everyone else had left.

I hadn't played with other children my age before. They seemed noisy, rough. I didn't know how to fight my way into the coveted playhouse or make friends with them. Unlike these children, I wasn't free in my body. Uneven surfaces, slopes, ice had to be negotiated, my legs frozen in terror. Biking and skating required fluidity. I could only watch, humiliated, an old lady in a child's body. Although I tried to minimize my "differences" to pass, the extent to which I lived in my body as a frozen shell was abundantly visible.

I remember waiting to answer the spelling quiz or the times tables, hoping I would get it right, fearing humiliation. My printing was smudged and messy. Pleased I could read like the other children, it quickly became my salvation, a way to live requiring only inactivity and solitary silence. I could live out all my desires without making a mistake, being laughed at or punished. For once there was only one message (not two or three) to decipher and negotiate. Through books I could think, feel and know I was alive. This has shaped who I have become, my "normal".

Writing was a problem. Like my mother, it seemed to require routine. I would sit and wonder how, in a sentence or a paragraph or a page, I could convey the wholeness, the beauty of what I could see in my mind. Each sentence seemed to negate or deny part of that picture. With the shattering of a sense of self before I had language, it is not surprising that expression presented a puzzle. Who was left to weave meaning between the shattered parts? Expression could also penetrate the mask of the terrorised child who knew too much. My survival depended on her disguise. I thought much and wrote little.

Church

Church was important in my God-fearing family. Welsh choral music is rooted in Protestant hymns. Our local church had a stained glass window of Jesus which said "I stand at the door and knock". I would wonder what I had to do to make that happen. Later I was enraged that even with God "who loved me" I was left to do all the work. His love didn't make a difference to the conditions of my life.

> When I was three I was put in a pine box that sat in an underground pit. It was dark down there. Bugs crawled on the sides of the pit. They said it was for my own good. I told myself that if I was careful not to touch the sides of the box, I wouldn't have to know where I was. When I wake up now, I find myself back in that same eerie stillness, staring at the ceiling. My wrists and ankles lie crossed, remembering the ropes that tied them.

> When the lid of the box came down, the last ray of light would disappear. Before the nails were pounded into the lid and I was abandoned, I would flip onto my side, seeking the comfort of the fetal position, holding my sense of life silently, deep inside, away from what was happening to me.

Later, when I attended a church youth group, the janitor befriended me, wanting me to sit on his lap. I fled. He wanted to explain. I withdrew. My childhood world was one of terror, disconnection, obedience and withdrawal, as well as regular routines, respectable manners, stories and music.

Solidifying The Mask

When I was nine I lay in bed one night and decided I was going to be first in my class. Over the next two years this happened. Learning came easily to a disciplined captive. The grubbiness and confusion of my earlier school years appeared to be left behind. Following my parents' example, my mask of competence, of niceness, froze into place. Hiding any imperfections, questions and doubts from others became my work.

My parents' expectations – that their children demonstrate impeccable manners, friendliness and concern for others – enhanced the mask. We were to be "better" than other people. Born in the more affluent period of my parents' life, their lessons in economy were augmented by trips to good restaurants, the ballet, the symphony. Ease in more polished environments added credibility to the mask. The mask, like my mother's routine, helped me function and forget.

When I was twelve, lessons in the dangers of letting the mask slip began. One of my sisters was admitted to hospital and given electroshock treatments for depression. She was at home caring for two young children when she started to cry and couldn't stop. At about the same time, one of my aunties spent a summer sitting in our garden in an unexplained state of collapse. Later, right after I married in my early twenties, my father spent months in hospital, anxious and depressed.

The mask took work and left me curiously unconnected to the world around me. The idealism of the sixties resonated with the longing of my hidden self. I was left mostly untouched by fashion, rock music, experiments with drugs, sex, the growing women's movement, communal living.

All this required being noticed, which was dangerous. I could not risk very much feeling or sensation beyond the confines of the mask. Sometimes I think it was musicals, with their hope of deliverance through romantic love, that kept me going.

I made a couple of friends and had many acquaintances. I was content with companionship, unable to risk exploring my interests in the world. Without risk-taking, mistakes and experiments, I did not learn to act on my desires, to sort out my differences from others and to jostle to create a place for myself in the world. I stayed in the safety of captivity behind a mask of others' expectations and what I saw as the safest way to negotiate the world. On the surface I looked normal: part-time work, university education, marriage, two children, comfortable home. Like in my mother's life, marriage and family were primary in the choices I made.

Under the surface lay inexplicable sadness and rebellion. I didn't feel part of how other people lived, and always wanted to be set slightly apart in how I dressed, what I thought or did.

Living Family Now
In March and April, 1997, my oldest sister has again become very ill. For twenty-five years I have minimized contact with this sister. Knowing she terrifies me and will never acknowledge the realities of my incest history, I have

not involved myself in her life or her care. Another sister stays with me when she comes to spend time with my oldest sister. These visits rip up my fragile present and fling me back into the past. In spite of my struggle, I rarely say no when she asks to stay. This refusal would deny my affection and cross some boundary of family acceptance I am unwilling to transgress.

With my oldest sister's illness, the family rallies around. Because of my sister staying in my house, I have some contact with other family members. Although all my siblings know about my incest history, through a letter I sent to them several years ago, there is no conversation with me about my lack of involvement. On the surface, everyone is pleasant. I come out of these encounters feeling confused, lonely and guilty. Revisiting these conversations, I begin to see their indirect, angry barbs. My sense of what is possible in my life shrinks back into the family mold of caring for others. Although I am diminished, I dig in my heels, not wanting to lose my incest history, my moments of feeling alive and connected, the trust I have built and the possibilities for tomorrow, under the blanket of family denial.

The Double-Edged Gifts of Normativity
The positioning of the incested family as dysfunctional, as "other" than "normal" families, erases the impact on the survivor of all the daily ways that incest families maintain social norms. I am aware of and grateful for the legacies which allowed us, as a family, and me, as an individual, to continue. I learned a strength of will from them and a capacity to hope some day things would be different. Love of music and well-expressed thoughts nurtured me. I received enough physical care, teaching in acceptable behaviour, and moments of affection to establish the habits of a life. My parents stressed education and encouraged me to think. In addition to my experiences of incest, the strength and power of these legacies shaped me and continue to bind me to my family. If these legacies bring pain, they also bring a sense of belonging and familiarity, connection to things I have loved as long as I have been alive.

This family legacy is a double-edged sword. It allowed me to establish a life that looked very similar to the people around me and helped sustain me in the horror living just below the surface of my life. It also makes it difficult to grasp and articulate the continued exploitative family patterns that are painful and alienating. I have no way of knowing whether being part of other families is as hurtful and confusing as being part of my own family; whether other families are as devoted to maintaining normativity through denial as my own.

My confusion with respect to family is also generated by my investments in behaving as a respectable female adult who meets her responsibilities toward family and the world with politeness and decorum. Bass &
Davis ask survivors to focus on how they feel during and after visits with
family and on what happens during the visit. They encourage survivors to
negotiate their needs with family members as a separate adult individual,
without acknowledgement of the investments survivors may have in
dominant social discourses about family and being a woman (1988).

While their questions clarify my feelings, they do not seem to solve my
dilemma. I, like my family, remain invested in the dictates of respectability,
in which women family members help care for their vulnerable members.
Ill and aging members require care; my house is needed as a place for my sister to stay. So I provide somewhere to sleep and pay the price of contact with
family after my sister leaves. Although I have minimized my involvement, to
refuse help is to refuse my formation as a respectable family member and
mature adult. It may also suggest that they may not be worthy of my care;
that I have positioned myself as "too good" for them. My refusal also entails
a possible unmasking of their respectability as well[14].

This is a very difficult place to hold. Acceptance by my family requires
me to hold my silence and to participate fully in the care of my oldest sister.
If I choose acceptance by them, I choose numbness and the loss of my
incest history. My refusal to do this leaves me open to indirect expressions
of anger, moments of unexpected coldness. Part of me longs to shatter my
family's denial through on-going confrontation and demand for accountability. I am deflected from taking this approach by its disrespect for the
ways my family copes with their pain, its futility and its "childishness". My
investment in behaving as a respectable and mature adult is as much a part
of me as my despair after my sister's visit. Within the dictates of respectability,
denial of the incest itself, denial of my vulnerability by my family and to
some extent my denial of my own vulnerability reverberate. My family's
requirements of me as a mature respectable woman, reinforced through
social norms, depend on this erasure and silence.

Respectability Creates Some Possibility of Family

In a family full of a silent history, the work of maintaining respectability
through adhering to social norms actually provides a vehicle to negotiate
the quagmire of rage, grief and despair that incest violation brings. Rather
than relate to one another honestly, we behave respectably. Looking at dysfunctional families from a psychological and relational point of view, Stiver

describes "how children learn how to stay out of relationships while behaving as if they are in relationships" (1990; Pt II:2). Strategies used include:

> 1) various forms of emotional disengagement which includes ... dissociative states as well as the use of substances which numb affect 2) role playing which refers to assuming a persona which seems adaptive and appropriate, but is not experienced by the person as authentic and 3) the replication of old interactions and family dynamics which are compelling and unrelenting. (1990:2)

My affection for family members and my desire for authentic relationships with them is layered by a history of learning and using all the strategies Stiver describes to stay out of and in relationship with them. Given the history of secrets within the family, hearing how they feel underneath their social mask terrifies me as does my own vulnerability with them. None of us have sufficient experience in relating cleanly to one another to take this risk. Our only hope of contact is through behaving respectably towards one another.

Breaking these patterns through honesty and direct negotiation would risk personal exposure and destroy the familiar fabric of my family. As painful and isolating as that can be, it also feels like home. This sense of familiarity, and my longing for "family", draws me back time after time, until I am wounded and withdraw once again.

Respectability Creates Silence

The parameters of respectability which create some possibility of relationship among my siblings now was taught by my parents. We were raised according to the dictates of white, middle-class WASP respectability and my parents insisted we behave accordingly. This respectability included an orderly structured household with three square meals, clean clothes, regular bedtimes; insistence on homework being done and on polite ladylike behaviour; attendance at church; the occasional trip to a movie or a concert. If I woke in the morning dissociated and too ill from the aftertaste of sperm to eat breakfast, there was no vehicle to name that experience as different from other children's. I just took crackers to eat at recess and fought down my nausea walking to school.

Adams describes the post-war era when I was a child as a time in which social values placed new emphasis on the family:

In this context having a family became a social marker of social belonging, of conformity to prevailing standards. It was a sign of maturity and adulthood, of one's ability to take on responsibility. (1994:58)

This is the "Leave It To Beaver" family, with mother at home producing well-adjusted children, and father at work. Family life became increasingly insular, the source of satisfaction for individual member's needs. Communism and sexual deviancy became the enemies against which strong families provided a buttress by building strong moral characters. At the same time, the post-war rise of psychology as a discipline created standards of "normal"development against which children were measured and the family's success implied (Adams, 1994:173). Breaking out of their denial would have cost my parents their social standing within the community, their sense of being competent adults, and the potential success of their family as measured by their children's achievements.

The impact of these discourses on my life as a child was to reinforce my conformity and silence my differences. For the most part, I participated in the work of my family to maintain the appearance of family success and minimize or hide any differences I may have felt from social norms. The encouragement within school to conform to their standards required the same performance of myself as my parents did. With a rocky enough hold on life, I would not risk breaking my silence, particularly in a social climate that had not yet publicly acknowledged the existence of childhood sexual abuse. If normativity is the lens through which families are seen, then it seems ironic that the family portrait as a social site of moral character-building was a place of immorality, horror, betrayal and pain for me and many other children.

My parents' emphasis on respectability, reinforced throughout my childhood, was probably compounded by their mixed-class positioning. I remember my mother telling me of a public health nurse twenty years earlier questioning my family's nutritional habits because my two oldest sisters were underweight for the "norm". She felt stung that their genetic inheritance of tiny bones could leave her open to questioning her adequacy as a mother. My mother's middle-class background and my father's ambition left them striving towards middle-class respectability in which their actions would not be subject to public scrutiny. The appearance of a middle-class life was constructed by my mother's disciplined economizing. Tuned to my parents' feelings for the sake of my survival, I registered my mother's fear of class censure and I live out her uneasiness in the raising of my own children within a financially constrained middle-class context (Miller, 1981).

As long as respectable families can maintain socially-defined parameters for physical care, financial stability and behavioural norms for its members, they will not be subject to public scrutiny. This impacts on the visibility of childhood sexual abuse. In their 1994 study of the processing of child sexual abuse cases, Gunn & Linden found that "many of the [reported] cases involved families who had multiple social problems" (107). Childhood sexual abuse is more likely be to "discovered" in situations where the family's capacity to hold its class respectability is already crumbling.

However, in middle-class families where mothers have tried to support their children's disclosure, the judicial system has not reinforced their actions. In her report on recent cases in which mothers entered into protective custody battles with their husbands after their children's disclosure, Armstrong found the judicial system frequently questioned the mother and protected the father:

> Mother after mother after mother, many of them with the self-view of post feminists – MBAs, teachers or professors, paediatricians, even attorneys, who believed the main battles had been won – found her life abruptly transformed, her career derailed, as she simply did what she believed society would support her in doing: believed her child and attempted to act to protect him or her ... And – with two or three exceptions among the hundreds of women whose cases I would follow over the next years – each of them lost custody, and not infrequently all visitation, most often to the alleged abuser. (1994: 134)

Alice Miller also documents the disbelief within the judicial system that accompanies accusations against respectable men. Because these men cannot be responsible, mothers and children are examined for their culpability. The child's trust is once again betrayed, this time by the futility of speaking (1990).

Criminal convictions are no easier to obtain than protective custody arrangements. In their study of the processing of child sexual abuse cases Gunn and Linden found that "the filtering out of reports at the police/Crown/court levels accounted for the termination of 71 per cent of the cases." (1994:106) Reasons for this include "the long delays of complaint, lack of corroboration and the Court's suspicion of children's evidence" (1994: 107).

When protective action was taken, Gunn and Linden found that the victim "was as likely as not to be removed from the home after disclosure" (1994: 107). Consigned to the social margins of child protection through the loss of their status as a respectable family member, children who speak out risk an uncertain future based on the availability and types of placements (Armstrong, 1993). They risk the anger of family members who don't want their respectability jeopardized, responsibility for their denial and inaction recognized or their economic support lost (Miller, 1990).

Respectability holds intact a complex web of class and gender power relations. These, in turn, influence who is perceived as credible, whose life is fundamentally altered by disclosure and who hides silently behind the walls of respectability.

The Respectable Dysfunctional Dichotomy

Rather than understand a family in which incest occurs as "other" from the norm of respectable families, the feminist analysis of the web of power and privilege within families places incest on a continuum of oppression of women and children within families. The sexual objectification of children and females within the family as possessions of their husbands and fathers, as well as the female responsibility to care for family members, create the conditions of oppression and possibility for incest (Kaschak, 1992; Jacobs, 1994). Within this context, there is little accountability for the actions of privileged male family members.

The separation made between "respectable" families and "dysfunctional" families in which violence occurs discourages accountability from the men who may be closest in our lives – our fathers, brothers, husbands and sons. Breaking the dichotomy between respectability and dysfunction would allow the question to surface of how our love, thoughts, actions and desires may be perpetuating violence and disguising power inequities. Acknowledging the oppression continuum within all heterosexual families requires grappling with the investments laid down by social norms of respectability.

The privileging of male interests and desires within the family and the powerlessness and dismissal of women results in a loss of relationship between female family members (Kaschak, 1992; Jacobs, 1994). What I needed from my mother, in addition to protection, were strategies for living as a strong authentic woman in a male-dominated world. What I got from her victimization reinforced my sense of powerlessness at the hands of my father (Jacobs, 1994). While I am angry at her actions and the ways her life reinforced images of women's oppression for me, I am also left to find recourse for my father's implicit entitlement to my body however I can. The therapeutic discourses of dysfunction which are predominant in incest writing maintain oppression by locating this struggle over the rights to my body as an individual, rather than a collective, endeavour (Armstrong, 1994; Alcoff & Gray, 1993; Tal, 1996).

Respectability brought coping mechanisms and sufficient social approval for my actions for me to survive. It continues to shape my relationships with family. In the end, I live somewhat outside ideal social norms regarding families. Every holiday, every change within the family, requires negotiating that difference. Feelings of love, the desire for connection, a sense of duty and obligation are weighed against the pain, fear, anger and sadness that family also brings. Developing traditions and relationships with people whom I trust provides an alternative to the dictates of family holidays as well as mutual support and affirmation.

What some lament as the social decline of family life and family values may also be seen as a struggle out of oppressive conditions by women now more able economically to support themselves and their children and so offer protection. The economic, emotional, physical and intellectual independence of women is key in ending the normative dominance of fathers in families. The lessening of the respectable family as predominant social norm creates greater possibilities for social perceptions to shift. The power of the father to access his daughter's body would therefore be recognized as abuse and would be fundamentally opposed.

Chapter 4

UNDER THE MALE GAZE

It is the very ordinariness of these activities; a weekend away, sitting at a baseball game, in a hockey arena, watching a snowball fight that make the lessons of these stories so difficult to unravel and accept, and so easy to blame myself for overreacting and not speaking up.

As the parent of a son, I have accompanied him to many activities and sat watching as he participated. It is not surprising I have come to see these activities as reproducing normative masculinity. I find it unsettling, however, that I can also see how ordinary, unseen acts of everyday violence are interwoven in the activities through which my son is becoming a man. I have strong, visceral reactions: surprise, longing, anger and fear associated with much of what I have seen.

The current therapeutic literature on incest perceives these reactions in terms of being "triggered"; a moment when past trauma intrudes on present day life, bringing strong emotions of terror, rage, or grief (Herman, 1992). The therapeutic goal is to gain sufficient insight into past trauma and practice to control these moments (Bass & Davis, 1988). Because my terror and rage are "inappropriate", or pathological, according to social norms for the activity, my reaction, and not the social relations to which I am reacting, becomes the site requiring change.

This articulation of how past trauma lives within the present reflects part of my experience of watching my son participate in his activities. Although being "triggered" is viewed as a "problem", it is also an invaluable, if costly, way to see through the blinders of ordinary life to underlying social relations of power and privilege. Within a psychological framework, the questions his activities raise are confined to my identity as an incest survivor. How my locations as a feminist, lesbian, mother and woman may interact with being an incest survivor are disregarded. Unpacking the contradictions within these sites of my experience presents a more complex understanding of an incest survivor's everyday experience.

Much of what preoccupies me within these stories is the performance of power within and through discourses of masculinity. Philip Corrigan maps this discursive range when he says:

> So what is constructed as masculinity, within common sense, confirmed and conformed at every turn, is a contradiction: on the one hand the desire to be a man in full plenitude – lonely, unattached, always strong, always able to do it, suddenly; on the other hand is a man responsible, reproductive of the values that count in the world, stability and monogamy . . . But there is, of course, a third element here, they have to do well . . . The trap is the denial of the free-ranging, moving shifting and singular concentration upon doing well within the male gaze. (1990: 282)

Within popular culture Corrigan's first version of masculinity is characterized by heroes like James Bond, John Wayne and Rambo; symbols of strength and physical action, masked self-reliance and virility in various class positionings. The second is that of a heterosexual husband and father upholding core social values and institutions. James Stewart in "It's a Wonderful Life" for example.[15] These contradictory positions are difficult for a male child to learn in order to position himself correctly according to socially-defined gendered norms (Davies, 1989). Maintaining acceptance, which is conditional on performance, creates on-going work.

In broad strokes, Kaufman defines the performative norms of masculinity when he says "masculinity means being in control, having mastery over yourself and the world around you. It means taking charge" (1993:28). Accepting rules and hierarchy, learning to perform and suppress feelings are all part of gaining mastery and control. Homophobia defines the boundary of intimacy among males (Kaufman, 1993; Messner, 1992) and violence supports its discourses of domination (Abbott, 1993). Just as access to power and privilege varies for men across race and class positionings, so will the expression of the tenets of masculinity.

None of this comes without a price. Jackson describes the costs of masculine discourses in which performance is based on mastery and control:

> The tension between the power I felt in the world of work . . .
> and the constant sense of wobbliness and precariousness in my

emotional life finally came to a head in my forties ... My previous shaky attempts to achieve a confirming performance, as a man precarious within his conventional masculinity, eventually collapsed into physical breakdown ... What I learned from it was that I couldn't go on imposing my conscious will on my feelings and bodily experiences and that I had to learn, however painfully, how to bring my feelings and my head together again. (1990:13)

The split men experience reflects a social public-private divide as well as an interior fragmentation. The permission men experience to be vulnerable in personal relationships pivots on their domination of women, and the constitution of their manhood as invulnerable. Within this contradictory position in personal relationships, "men are set-up to embody and enact violence against women" (Corrigan, 1990:283).

As I begin to unravel my incest history and learn to live with my terror, rage and grief, my interest in these stories reflects my questions of how to take up positions of power within the world. As I watched my son, for example, I had a multitude of responses to masculine positionings. When my son was asked to go on playing baseball in spite of the physical shock from a collision at home plate, it reverberated for me with the conditions of incest captivity I was struggling to undo. At the same time, I was enchanted as I watched him learn physical mastery, knowing that with the damage of my incest history it will be unlikely for me to gain these skills. As a feminist and an incest survivor, I felt compelled to address the subtle overlay of violence in his activities and found this difficult to express. Always, in these stories, I grapple with judgement about not performing adequately under the male gaze. Unravelling the layers of ordinary life, I explore the impact of normative discourses of masculinity on my son and myself.

Cub Camp

Without knowing it we were learning that masculinity involved learning to "discipline" our bodies and our unruly emotions. It required learning and accepting relationships of power and hierarchy. (Kaufman, 1993:61)

I think that I can just go and participate in something. Over and over I learn about the impact of incest on my everyday life. It is never as simple as just going. There is so much to pay attention to, to negotiate now.

57

In September, 1991 when my son was eight and had been in Cubs for a few months, I agreed to pick up the boys after a weekend at Cub camp. I liked how the Akela, or leader, acknowledged the boys' work at the closing and the sense of community that seemed to be there. Seeing my interest, the Akela encouraged me to come again. The next year I decided my contribution to Cubs would be to help at the fall camp. I did not realize how long this weekend would be.

Friday night, when we arrive, I'm glad to be told what to do and that I know how to do the badge work that I will teach (putting up a tent). Intimidated by the new situation and the number of men, I automatically slip into my family survival mode. I want to be helpful and to fit in. We are given thick binders on Cub camp in which even the menus are planned. The women are not responsible for putting the boys to bed. I am delighted. I retreat happily to bed with a book.

Saturday morning, only my roommate, who is another lesbian mother, and I have slept well; we have the good mattresses. At breakfast several of the boys seem upset, uncomfortable. I reassure, smile and mother. The Akela tells the boys that there is lots of food and choices if they hate what they are served. This would not have occurred to me. I'm glad he has this kind of insight. No one but the cooks are allowed in the kitchen. I feel kicked out of my domain and dislike having to wait for more coffee. In a male domain women usually have power in the kitchen, access to food. Here I lack even that.

The badge work begins. I like the contact with each small group or "six". I am expected to "mark" each group member on their enthusiasm and efficiency, to establish a hierarchy between the groups through competition. The "best" group will receive an award at the end of the weekend. By mid-morning some of the boys seem restless with the activities, preferring to do their own thing. In their uniforms they seem to act out masculine caricatures: the pip squeak with the karate chop, the bully, the non-conformist who describes the chapel as mystical. Conformity and participation are stressed. Those who have "trouble" should be helped by the others.

By Saturday afternoon I'm bored. I'm only needed as an extra set of adult hands. I dislike that my autonomy is being taken away and that I'm not being given a task. I want to be off on my own. The other lesbian mother feels the same way, which helps. Several people comment on my "Stop Violence Against Women" button left on my coat from International Women's Day. I'm unsure how to take their comments, what a public mention of male violence means in this environment, how I could be targeted. In the past,

I believed my safety depended on being invisible except in well-known, predictable environments. While waiting for the next group the Cub pack next door scatters the tent parts I left rolled up on the ground. I'm disillusioned with the "good citizen" rhetoric of Cubs. In the speed and silence with which they collect the scattered tent parts, it is clear they understand that one of the rules of respectability is to not touch other people's stuff. Without the presence of a visible authority figure, the boys behave in a destructive way. I, as a woman (read: mother) have to call them on it and get them to clean it up. I blame myself for not knowing better, for being too trusting.

Before dinner I accompany the boys to the obstacle course, grateful I'm not required to climb the thirty-foot wall. One boy says he has to go to the bathroom. I accompany him. He is upset at having pooped his pants. The paths are confusing. I reassure him and think about my own son, who says he'd rather hold his poop than use the outhouse. When I offer to take the flak for him using the indoor toilets, forbidden to the boys during the day, he refuses. Obedience to the rules established by male hierarchy is more important than the needs of his own body.

When we return to the main building, five men are sitting in the kitchen drinking beer and talking. I tell the boy what to do and send him off. I'm told I'm not allowed in the kitchen, but I can come in if I drink a beer. When I was young, I would have been flattered by this invitation, this inclusion. Now being one of the boys is not something I want or value. This leaves me feeling out of place, without an automatic role to slip into. I ask if one of them will check on the boy. The worst of the chauvinists (a father of four boys) does. Another man says "You prefer eight-year-olds to us, eh?" Terrified by the undercurrent of combined sexuality and threat, I leave.

The boys look better at dinner. I move from boredom to mild hostility. As the group comes together, my caretaking is needed less. There is more room for me to feel what I am really feeling. I don't find the men's jokes funny. My son is told twice to freeze and return to his seat when he doesn't follow the rules. The male chauvinist says he has wine and treats. We, the adults, are to come over to the men's cabin once the boys are in bed.

Before bed we are told we must watch a traditional game. It turns out to be an initiation trick on new parents. Everyone gets very wet and appears to enjoy the fun. Neither myself nor the other lesbian is picked for initiation. I think that is interesting. We watch a racist and sexist movie called "Sergeant Swell", a long-standing tradition in this troupe. I had hoped to get away by myself and read during the film but was told to sit. If I refuse I might cause trouble and be reprimanded, so I obey.

Once the boys are in bed, I agree to accompany the other lesbian mother to the "party" in the men's cabin. I won't go without you, she says. We have no choice. Of course we had choices. We could go and maintain the facade of pleasant cooperation or we could refuse and risk censure. For all women risking censure by men includes risking violence (Kaschak, 1992). As an incest survivor this possibility is particularly heightened.

The talk! They talk of the homosexual at the local senior public school with open sores on his face who had a nervous breakdown and talked about his lover in class. When I talk about our kids needing gay role models, the talk stops, then resumes on the other side of my blip.

They recall being "straightened out" as boys through having their knuckles and bottoms slapped, swimming naked in the school pool. Stories of other Cub camps are told, dunking one child's head in a toilet and trussing up another like a pig for three hours. His father had walked out saying "do what you want with him." The women are told our boys behave better when we are not there. One man tells his kids he's not their dad when they are at camp. The father of one of the boys who was upset at breakfast is here. I feel numb. There is permission here to be violent in the name of toughening up. I wonder if they'd say I "asked for it" as a baby.

The talk becomes racist. The need for Canadians to adopt the Americans' melting pot philosophy. Menorahs in the hall are fine but we should be allowed to sing Christmas carols. Akela reads, he is not participating. A Jewish father downs five beer in a row. As we return to our cabin, one of the men tells us that someone will be kidnapped. Afraid of becoming the victim, my roommate experiments with placing a chair under the doorknob.

Morning brings a search for a 'kidnapped child' while breakfast is prepared. We trudge through the woods carrying the ransom, a bag of Fudgeo cookies. Why is reproducing violence, threat of bodily harm, fun? I am tired of playing along. As always, I'm worried about humiliating myself. This time it's by being too numb and scared to feel my legs as they negotiate the steep slope.

At the end of the ravine there is a rope to swing over the river. I hang back, wanting to risk trying it but fearing humiliation. Longing for brilliance, I end up wet like the other adults. Fear and shame creep under my laughing and playing along. By not performing with effortless competence (like a man), the shadow of fighting off my father with all I had and losing night after night is with me again, in another "failure". As one of the leaders, a much-teased heavy man, crosses on foot, I call to the boys to come, wanting to distract them.

The morning drags on with a long soccer game. I watch in disbelief as the men, determined to win, play all-out against the boys who are much smaller. They call to me to join in. One boy gets hurt and lies shocked and in tears. Those who don't play don't cause trouble. Even the other lesbian mother seems to fit in this morning in a way I can't.

We pack up. My relief is enormous. Akela asks me to supervise lunch. I have trouble. The boys are supposed to raise their hands and not get up when they want something. I know crowd control is important in large groups, but this is ridiculous. Why are we not teaching them inner control? Why must all their control be external? I am half-hearted and uncomfortable.

Clean-up begins. The men's washroom is so smelly I can't believe we didn't clean it yesterday. I avoid the hints about the men's cabin. I say good-bye to the women and wave vaguely to the men. My car drives funny. I have a flat. I know there are several men behind me. I ask one if he will be my white knight? As I say it I can't believe that I, for all my feminist rhetoric, would stoop so low. They fix the tire quickly. I help as much as I can. I thank them, aware of my old car against their flashy new ones. I don't feel very successful.

As I drive home, away from danger, my numbness fades and my feelings return. I am angry, terrified and powerless. In this well of emotion I lose my ability to express what I know is wrong. I blame myself for not intervening. Maybe I'm over-reacting? I can't find my ground or my authority. The little I say to people about the weekend does not resonate for them beyond their question, "What did I expect?"

I tell my son's father what happened. He told me wonderful stories of Cub camp when I first met him. He said yes, they always tied up a new boy and left him in the woods on the first afternoon. Where was this story when we decided to put son in Cubs? Does he not see how terrifying this could be for the boy? Has he just not thought about it? Is he the same as other men who think this is alright? I feel now I must justify the decision to put our son into Cubs. I struggle alone to understand and articulate what is wrong with this community activity that has a long and honourable tradition.

A year later, I don't go to Cub camp although my lesbian friend does. She tells me it was different. One of the parents objected to "Sergeant Swell" so strongly it may not be shown next year. The badges were kidnapped this year rather than one of the boys. I still feel powerless and confused. Does it really make a difference to kidnap a bag of badges? The participation in extortion is still present. One parent seems to have got the message across. Why couldn't I do that? I am left feeling angry and impotent.

The connections between the activities of Cub camp and dominant discourses of masculinity are clear. For the boys, living in a hierarchical structure, performing as a team member under a leader, and competing individually and as a team, exposed them to situations for proving themselves "manly" as well as providing them with desired participation in the world of men. The father who denied his role as father to his son while at Cub camp encouraged his son to perform without emotional support. The overlay of kidnapping and extortion linked the attainment of masculinity to discourses of violence. Because the men reproducing these lessons appear to live their lives at the stable end of the masculine continuum, the importance of mastery and control for all versions of masculinity can be seen. Physical and emotional control within this overlay of violence are equally important for performing as the father and as the warrior, or so it seems.

What is perhaps more complex in this story are the ways these discourses of masculinity framed my participation and my experience. One of the subtleties of my experience at Cub camp was feeling my power completely displaced. I was away from home, in physical proximity to more men than I am likely to interact with over several months. I was living in a world in which I felt I could have no impact or influence. I couldn't even go into the kitchen for another cup of coffee. On the first night I was handed a binder outlining how Cub camp was to be done. My presence as a volunteer, an extra set of hands, not my thoughts and reactions, was all that was wanted of me within this hierarchical structure.

A second layer of my displacement relates to normative discourses regarding the parenting of boys. Silverstein & Rashbaum articulate the cultural importance of turning a boy over to his father, to the community of men in general, for socialization (1994:15). The lack of a father is often articulated as the reason why boys fail to achieve balanced and respectable masculine identities[16]. Mothers actively participate in this process of turning their sons over to their father and are blamed if their sons resist or do not achieve a sufficient "masculine" identity. Some of my confusion is the result of my own socially-constructed doubts about my knowledge and experience in parenting a boy.

A third layer relates to the active resistance and devaluing of the feminine throughout the weekend. Because masculinity is defined through a dichotomous relationship with the feminine (Benjamin, 1988), being a man leaves little room for qualities associated with women, such as relationship and nurturing. My vulnerability, through my inability to physically compete, and the fear bubbling under the surface, defined me clearly within a feminine framework and left me open to derision unless I acquiesced.

The effect of these displacements was that the women did not confront the men. Although some of the other women expressed their unhappiness with what was happening to one another, all of us "coped" and "helped" as best we could. In doing this we upheld the social norms for a weekend of adults supervising children and of our femininity. We played it safe. If the silence had been broken by the women, the men, in turn, might have been unwilling to disrupt their expectations of the weekend long enough to hear what was being said.[17] Clearly, the men were invested in the discourses of masculinity they were reproducing. The ways that we were displaced as women and mothers would become the arguments against what we were saying. This control over the dominant framework maintains male power and privilege.

The impact on me of this displacement was profound. As a feminist and a lesbian I felt compelled to address the implicit violence. As a mother I was reluctant to act and alienate my son when he clearly seemed to enjoy himself at Cubs. I wanted to wait and hope he would lose interest. This is, in fact, what happened. As an incest survivor, my inability to impact those in control, evident in the message of being an extra set of hands, threw me back into the captive conditions of the past with its obedience, terror, and futile angry rebellion.

What I longed for was not to become so undone by it all. I longed to take up a masculine identity like John Wayne, who would either shrug and walk away or blast them with three pithy sentences (since it is the 1990's). Academic Janet Jacobs, who has interviewed incest survivors, would see this as a survivor's over-identification with a perpetrator (the masculine). With the unravelling of my physical and emotional numbness through the process of recovering memory, I feel undone by my vulnerability and long for the inviolate male. Caught within the cultural dichotomies of male and female, weaving them together to feel, to live in my body, to hold strong boundaries and confront violence publically seems impossible.

My marginalized identities as lesbian, incest survivor and woman all stress the importance of breaking silence and challenging oppressive social relations. Knowing how other women's courage has supported my life, I feel obligated to participate in this work. This does not appear to be a simple task. Through the habit of silence from my childhood, I am left unable to accurately judge the degree of danger which speaking may entail within any particular set of social conditions. I am aware of how the knowledge resulting from my marginalized identities could be quickly pathologized and spill out in the objectification of myself and possibly my son. Within the narrative of Cub camp, in which the women are told by the men that their presence negatively affects their sons, there is no room to hear and receive knowledge of my lesbian, incest survivor, feminist identities. The only entry point is as someone seeking to disrupt, refuse or undermine the story[18]. Rather than take a stand and push the issues (which takes a certainty I rarely possess), my inclination is to want to talk about what's happening. Without a willingness to examine the investments – mine included – in the situation, it is relatively easy to dismiss what is being questioned. Pathologizing the individual who speaks up is one of the most prevalent ways power and privilege is maintained.

Acutely aware of my vulnerability, under the male gaze I judge myself as not living up to what I believe in, not performing adequately. It is also under their specific male gaze that I could have been judged if I did speak up. In staying within the complexity of my feelings, I fail to achieve rational control, the normative standard of the male gaze.

As the next story reveals, boys' performance as "men" goes on within the family home as well as with the local Cub pack. Although I am shocked by what I discover, I am also eager to join in.

Snowball Fight

In my son's lifetime there has never been as much snow as there is today, after a snow storm in December, 1992. He loves how it piles up on railings and covers signs. Watching him, I remember the enchantment of snowfalls, not the driving or shovelling, but making snowmen and angels, walking among huge drifts. The beauty and quiet of its presence.

By nightfall I'm tired by the unusual demands of the day. The children are crabby. I gratefully accept an invitation for dinner at the house of a neighbour and friend, looking forward to being nurtured. We arrive for pizza. There are extra kids, I enjoy the din, the sense of inclusion among many in a family that is not as conflicted for me as my own family of origin.

After dinner my friend's husband pours me a cognac. I relax in its warmth and his generosity. He and all the children disappear into a pile of winter clothes. It is time for war! I don't react to the implied violence of the game's name. I'm simply grateful that my children are carried along by the group and don't need my attention. My friend and I finish the clean-up and sit drinking tea, watching the activity. She talks about this game disintegrating when the big boys "forget" their strength and the little guys end up crying. I have heard this before from her and I'm puzzled by it. In the ordinariness of a leisurely evening and the familiarity of a family setting I understand as "safe", my antenna is at rest.

They spend a long time constructing huge walls of snow. Plastic recycling containers are soon full of snowballs. I watch, fascinated, having never seen a family playing like this. Snowballs start to fly. My daughter seems to be enjoying herself. I start to wonder where my son is.

My friend wants to go out. "For five minutes," she says. How excited they'll be if we come out too. We stand in the front yard making our basket of snowballs, giggling and planning our "attack". By now I am keen to take the risk and join in, wanting to expand beyond the confines of safe watching where I normally live. As usual, I am a little scared that I won't be able to handle it. But I want to be able to do what "normal" people do. My son comes around the corner from the back, crying and holding his eye. He turned around off-guard and received a snowball in the eye. In retrospect, I realize he received what I dreaded, that is more than he could handle.

But at the time, I am not sure what to do. He seems more angry than hurt. I don't want to stop and mother. I listen and say little, hoping he can work it out. At one point I start to make snowballs. He lets out a howl and I stop. My friend wonders if his eye is scratched and wants to have a look. He doesn't want anyone near it. She tells him to close it as it might feel better.

In the mud room we sit on the stairs while he cries and rages. I think of the hard week he has had, with a change of schools imminent. My friend comes in, saying her husband said my son seemed scared. I say I wouldn't be surprised. She goes and gets a washcloth for his eye which he accepts. I sit wondering why practical things like washcloths don't occur to me, slipping once again into self-blame.

Feeling guilty for resisting further caretaking, I say I want to play for a bit. He can come or stay in the house and play with one of the kids who has not ventured out. We will all be in soon, the fire is on. He decides to come with us. My friend tells him to hide in the fort when he needs to.

The snowball fight is very exciting. Mostly, I stay on the sidelines, more protected and able to modulate the amount of perceived danger, as well as my terror. I get the oldest boy on the neck, which leaves me feeling gleeful, guilty and scared of revenge. I receive enough snowballs to feel part of it. The oldest boy, a cousin, prances around delighted, strong enough to take the snowballs and watch out for the little boys. My son retreats crying, and shortly, swallows his tears.

The father and the oldest son, who is thirteen, walk up to each other with huge blocks of snow and crash like two titans. Shortly after, the thirteen-year-old approaches his ten-year-old brother. When the younger boy doesn't retreat, the older boy plows his face with snow. The ten-year-old rages and cries, unable to "take" the punishment of challenging a stronger "opponent". His father tells him not to wreck it for everyone else, to "get" his brother back or go into the house. The game ends shortly after with everyone wrecking the snow walls. When the ten-year-old continues complaining about his older brother, his father sends him to his room.

Their youngest son – unscathed throughout the snowball fight – and my son stay out for a long time after everyone else goes in. They play a slower version of a similar game. The little boy comes at my son with all his strength. My son does not retaliate or retreat. Neither is demolished or humiliated. Excited and happy, they run to make more snowballs. I am reminded of the nights after supper when my son and I push against each other, palm to palm, to feel our strength but not to overpower one another. This assertive experience of power brings me hope.

The snowball fight was a vehicle through which some male family members struggle over their place within the hierarchy. The boys took on the hierarchical framework as their own. Schwartz maintains that "the need to establish these hierarchies and to find one's place in them was an obsession for many boys, as struggles for security and power in concrete terms" (1993:164).

In the anthology *Boyhood, Growing Up Male,* many men describe their fear of humiliation and their ambivalence about participating in competitive struggle. Murray outlines the emotional dynamics boys experience:

> We learn from the culture that we're supposed to appear strong; not to let things bother us; not to give in to hurt or pain; not cry. So we bury the hurt, the pain, the anger, the shame – the stings of our boyhood. We forget about them. But when we find someone weaker than us, the buried feelings take their long awaited revenge. (1993: 51)

The boys in the middle age group had the hardest time in the snowball fight. Those who could compete successfully were fine. Those in the middle, testing their strength, competing for a place, got creamed by superior strength and became legitimate targets for aggressive retaliation. The code of masculine ethics to protect women and children as well as the lack of threat that they put forward, left the youngest son and the women outside the aggressive loop (Silverstein & Rashbaum, 1994).

Corrigan's articulation of the double-edged quality of families for men (a site where emotional nurturing is possible and domination must be maintained) is also present for boys (1990). Heterosexual families are a site of nurturing and care as well as a site of struggle to perform according to the dictates of masculinity. Activities valued by the family, the emotional withdrawal of mothers from their sons, the reactions of family members and the boy's responses to everyday events such as fights in the school yard, crying, dress up, physical contact all shape how a boy performs himself as masculine.

Within dominant tenets of mastery and self-control, the range of masculine identities from stable father to solitary hero allows for individual and class differences. Messner outlines the role of class in contributing to greater fluidity:

> ... boys from middle-class backgrounds developed their identities
> within a context that afforded them a wide range of options, and
> their family, educational, and peer group experiences tended to
> expand their awareness of these options. (1992: 68)

This range of acceptable masculine performance broadens the base of potential support and participation. Even women can perform well "as one of the boys" and gain recognition in the moment according to these standards. It is from this perspective that my desire to see "if I can take it" can be understood. By wanting to perform adequately, I uphold the tenets of masculinity.

I seem to live this story somewhere between motherhood and boyhood. The style of middle-class mothering that I conduct has been described by Walkerdine & Lucey (1989) as facilitative: I don't dictate to my son but provide a limited range of "choices" for him. By wanting to play I am attempting to throw off the passivity, the survival strategies of my incest childhood. I am still uncertain about my capacity to take care of myself. By choosing to play over staying with my son I reinforced masculine performance as desirable.

My son reacted strongly to what was happening. Perhaps his reference point of "normal" was based in other possibilities besides this competitive struggle. Although, by societal standards, my son lives in a "broken" home, the idea of alternative standards helps me to affirm the values in my present family. These values include an emphasis on cooperation and respect, and on direct, rather than indirect, verbal expression of feelings. My hope is that his version of masculinity will include capacities to recognize others as subjects of their own lives rather than as objects to be controlled.

> The upper classes appropriated existing sports and meanings of sports in ways that supported and then shaped the structure, rules, values and furthered their own interests.

> . . . the fact that sport was an exclusively male world made it seem natural to equate masculinity with competition, physical strength and skills. (Messner, 1992:10,31)

Baseball

This year, my son moved from the protectedness of T-ball – where no one catches, hits or runs with much accuracy – to baseball, where mistakes get noticed and skills are more important. Once again I romanticise his coaches as men who are not too competitive, who want to help boys develop their skills and enjoy playing. My son sits in the middle of the pack. He remembers the rules as he plays and throws quite well. I sit watching how exposed and visible he is and find myself worrying that he will be humiliated by some mistake. Even as I think it, I'm aware that this feeling is about me and the replaying of my history, and not about him. One father, a neighbour, moves about, barely able to watch, not wanting to utter a word when his son makes a mistake or doesn't pay attention.

Tonight my son slid unsuccessfully into home, scraping his leg and arm in a collision with the catcher. He was sobbing and shaking with shock. The coach and his assistant sat him down, wanting to examine him, without giving him time to recover and absorb the impact. I went over, placed my hand on his back and said, "Just give yourself a minute." I could feel the coaches' disapproval of my presence. After what seemed like a minute the coach said "Are you ready to go into left field, son? I really need you buddy or I wouldn't ask." Still shaking, my son got up, limped into left field and shortly regained his composure. As he did, I wondered what he learned from that.

Looking back, I think in that moment he learned to shut down his pain and feelings and carry on because the team needed him in order to win (Jackson, 1990; Messner, 1992). His desire to meet their demands of "normative boyhood performance" could result in his loss of emotional and physical connectedness. As I sat watching, engaged on a daily basis in slowly learning the difficult task of inhabiting a body that is not numb, the process of "toughening" him up stood out for me. I lost my connection to my body through victimization. My son may lose his in pursuit of masculine performance.

I am left to wonder about the role physical numbness plays in domination; is it easier to violate someone if your capacity to experience physical and emotional pain is reduced? Maintaining connectedness to the body and feelings seems like one of the first steps in undoing violence.

Both sexes are taught to control their bodies and feelings through their mind to attain their appropriate gender positionings. Boys are taught physical and emotional control over pain as part of performing male agency. Girls learn to focus their physical and emotional energy towards meeting the needs of others. The physical and emotional lessons survivors of sexual abuse learn include disintegration and dissociation. Controlling my fear leads not to the satisfaction of achievement as it may for boys, but to the dangers of dissociation, of not being present to what I am experiencing. Gendered positionings do not offer a model of the physical, emotional and mental integration for which I long. At the same time, the inviolate nature of masculine mastery and control draws me as a possible protection against my vulnerability.

Within my motherhood role, I raise questions about how my son is feeling following the game. My attempt to problematize his experience is drowned out by his investments in performing appropriately as a boy. My own inexperience with physical competition leaves me without any certainty about the degree of numbness between body and feelings in sports, without the authority to strenuously object. My inaction supports his development of an appropriate masculine performance and does not seriously challenge the potential dangers to my son's well-being and to perpetuating violence that learning physical and emotional numbness may entail. The same mixture of doubts, questions and investments carries on as our life together takes us to the hockey arena.

Hockey

We were allowed body contact and I loved it. It didn't have to do with sexuality and everything to do with power and with permission. It's a discovery of what your body can do and what it can be. That thump. That's power and it's something girls rarely get to experience . . . I now know that no matter how hard I try, I'll never be able to play the boys' game, the game of "pain equals respect". Truthfully, I don't even understand it. But I proved myself to the boys. Maybe next time they see a female hockey player, they won't underestimate her. (Kirzner-Roberts,1992:12,13,19,21)

In 1992, my son begins to play hockey in a league, after several years of hockey school. He is more interested in playing and wants to make the school team. Because close family friends encourage their boys to play, my son has had more than average contact with boys who play hockey.

I have resisted his playing, not wanting the "chore" of getting him there twice on the weekend and feeling ambivalent about the stories I have heard about hockey parents. With a car pool arranged to share the work and the early mornings, my objections are silenced.

I have been watching and listening for about a month now, taking in a completely new experience. I sit with a neighbour who talks of being flooded with happy memories of boyhood hockey when he enters an arena. Some of my own memories of popcorn, a fire and Hockey Night in Canada return as we watch the game. My knowledge of the rules warms up again.

I feel the magic, the quiet of the arena, the beauty of bodies moving easily, the sound of their blades, their doggedness in trying to get a goal. The boys come off sweating, pleased with themselves, full of the story of the game, what they did well, who screwed up. My neighbour's family has a tradition of stopping at the discount donut house next door, part of memories being created. As time goes on I struggle with the question of stopping for donuts, with saying no and yes, wanting an "exciting" alternative to the sugar high that spins me away from maintaining an embodied connection, and one that the children will accept.

I feel "Canadian" on hockey days, back in my father's stories of his boyhood playing on a frozen pond. I let go of my anger at professional hockey, the hype, the money, the fights, of people who prefer engaging with a winning team to engaging in their own lives.

I wonder how boys are formed through playing on a team. Do they learn to get the job done in spite of weaknesses? Watching, I long for the ease of the boys on skates gained through practice, their ability to use their bodies as they wish, without deliberate thought and fear; their courage to get in the middle of a play and fight for the puck. This physical mastery is linked for me, as an individual and within the culture, as a whole with agency and success (Messner, 1992; Jackson, 1990). Yet even without these social connotations, it seems beautiful in and for itself.

I feel shaken and overwhelmed after the boys' game today, back in the terror of my abuse. More parents are attending games as the season wears on. As the other teams improve, my son's team struggles more. Parents screamed today, focussed on winning at any cost. "Skate, skate, skate, Brian." "Get him, get him, get him," when one boy attempted a break away. "I'm not paying all this money for you to stand around," as the boys crashed in a bunch and tried to sort out sticks, arms and legs. It could have been slap-stick comedy. The parents around me, committed to competition and performance, did not see the humour. Hearing the edge at which they were poised, where the drive to succeed overrides everything, I became frightened, knowing well the costs of this furious desire when there is no referee to blow the whistle.

In my son's second hockey year, as the winter wears on, I wonder if my relationship with him is too shaped by activities that I endure, like hockey. I want fewer "shoulds" with both my kids, more life and engagement.

For his thirteenth birthday in 1995, my son wanted his friends to play a leisurely game of hockey on an indoor rink for an hour. One girl and twelve boys showed up, combining roller blading, figure skating, road and ice hockey. Down at bench level I watched their growing teenage bodies, exhilarated as they combined will, muscle, skill and desire for the sheer pleasure of it. I saw how practice over time creates confidence, the joy of accomplishment, of using your body well.

The survivor in me longs for the embodied sense of agency and confi-dence that I saw in my son and his friends for that hour. As someone engaged in reconnection with my body, being embodied is full of lyrical desire. A father who coaches hockey laughed and responded to this saying, "Philosophically you're right, but the fuel through the hard times out there is competition."

At hockey practice, in December, 1996, I am grateful just to sit at this busy time of year, comforted by the familiarity of being here. As I watch the boys proceed through the drills and listen to the coaches' comments, I see how entitlement intrinsic to privilege is being taught. Time is set aside on a regular basis for learning skills. Advice and encouragement are available. Most of all, the boys learn to survive being visible agents in a public arena. They are taught the discipline of practice, that with time and attention they'll acquire the skills to perform in a public place. This communicates a sense of entitlement which underlies class privilege.

There are seductive moments for me watching hockey at the arena. Moments when I see the physical, emotional and mental embodiment I seek.

Moments when I see the power of teamwork in achieving a goal. These are moments when I envision the possibility of this connectedness for myself and with others; moments before the realities of terror, frozenness and alienation reemerge.

For my son, the seduction is different. He talks about his enjoyment of the increasing physical contact, playing on the edge of the rules. He says "you wouldn't understand Mom, it's a guy thing." He is probably more focussed on the ice than at any other time. He wants to achieve a level of masculine performance so he can compete aggressively in arenas where violence is thinly disguised and externally controlled by the referee (Messner, 1992:68). His reference to this being "a guy thing" marks the gender boundary of my influence. Although I am aware of the consequences of aggressiveness once the referee has gone home, I am not part of the equation.

The teamwork which seduces me with its appearance of cooperative effort and equality is actually a highly stratified, competitive structure resonating with Foucault's discussion of discipline. The boys are learning to regulate their bodies in particular ways in order to be successful players and team members.[19] This regulation defines individual responsibility in terms of fulfilling a role and reproduces individual inequity as part of the system. There is the strong normative behaviour of positional play required, leaving the individual player blameless for the outcome as long as he has fulfilled his defined responsibilities. At the same time, there is the possibility of recognition for exceptional skill or drive. I wonder if my son's enjoyment comes from both the recognition he obtains from performing adequately under the rules and from the possibility of further recognition for exceptional play. The fleeting nature of this recognition requires him to hone his skills and continually reproduce his masculine performance. Teamwork is achieved by the coordination of individual performances rather than by the interconnectedness between players.

Pride Day

In 1996, my son is given the opportunity to work at the Second Cup coffee shop in the heart of Toronto's gay and lesbian ghetto on Pride Day. My neighbour, who works there, says they are desperately shorthanded. My son is keen to do it. He is interested both in earning money and having the opportunity to learn something new. I am delighted, as he has never agreed to accompany me on Pride Day, although his sister has. They have had similar exposure to anti-racist, anti-sexist, anti-homophobia education through an alternative school. Although I notice a softening in him, he seems much less affected by this teaching than my daughter. We go downtown together to watch some of the parade before he begins work. I want him to have some exposure to the sheer numbers of people before he starts. As we wind our way through the crowd, he attracts a lot of interest from gay men. He is a good-looking kid. Part of me wants to wrap him in cellophane so he can't be touched, and part of me admires the blatancy with which these men own their sexual desire. He seems bored stiff as we watch the parade. He is less able to get into the festive spirit than my daughter the year before. He tells me S&M is gross. Although perhaps for different reasons, I agree.

Late that night, we sit on the steps of the Second Cup. He has finished working. The interest of other men in him continues as he wolfs down another dinner. He tells me about learning the espresso machine, hauling bags of ice in the heat, how nice they were to him, how much his feet hurt. Several men asked him if he was gay. He says he told them that his mother is lesbian. "Oh, so you don't hate us old faggots then, eh?" said one, as the man bent down and kissed my son on the cheek. He tells me of seeing men French kissing. "It was ok mom, it was just the first time I'd seen it." He repeats how much he dislikes the S&M scene, revealing his investment in the stable Jimmy Stewart end of the masculine continuum. Other than a statement he once made that all his close friends have lesbian mothers, I still don't know very much about how he "manages" his mother being lesbian.

As I step back from this story, I see my son's participation in Pride Day requires him to negotiate a complex space between social discourses on heterosexual masculinity and a personal connection to his lesbian mother. Proximity to the gay community could potentially leave him open to questions about his masculinity from other men. Because masculinity is defined in relation to a misogynist dichotomy of "sissy, pansy, fairy" (Seidman, 1993), it is not only his sexual orientation that could be questioned but his basic definition as male. I wonder how much of the attention he attracted was the result of gay men pushing this boundary?

As a lesbian mother, my responsibility to raise a son includes challenging misogyny and homophobia. My ability to do so depends on my own capacity to maintain a critical edge within daily life. I am constantly wondering what I am not seeing, what I am replicating (King, 1997). In addition to this critical edge, as an incest survivor I feel a responsibility to teach non-violent strategies. All this requires me to constantly grapple with questions, with a sense of unease reflected throughout these stories. My inability to maintain a sense of rational control, wondering if I am doing "enough" enfolds with the incest survivor's sense of self-blame. However, it also reflects the normative evaluative standard of the male gaze. While I do play an important role in my son's development, it would be naive not to acknowledge the power of what he learns about being masculine from normative social relations surrounding us both.

There is hope in the lesbian community that "our" generation of sons will be different, through their daily exposure to mothers who are emotionally available, have agency and live out different relationships to the polarities of masculinity and femininity. The depth of individual investments this chapter reveals suggests how bringing this hope into reality requires on-going reflection on everyday practices.

Perhaps the place where I have taken the most direct public role with regard to shaping my son's masculinity has been through finding alternative educational spaces in which he can experience different expectations regarding himself as male. Because of our location in a white middle-class urban environment, there is access to alternative schools that will challenge the "isms" governing social normativity and nurture possibilities for cooperation and creativity. These schools potentially broaden the range of acceptable masculine performance.

While I search for environments that can do this and am grateful when I find them, my privilege does not create a solution to the narrowing of masculinity towards control, performance and acceptance of hierarchy.

A More Complex Understanding

Exploring the intersections between my identities as feminist, lesbian, mother and incest survivor results in a more complex understanding of how my individual investments shape my behaviours and responses than an exploration from a psychological perspective would. Uncovering how dominant social discourses interact with experience offers greater insight into survivors' lives than the psychological position which views survivors as struggling to attain normativity. What I find particularly interesting is how the situations in these stories, which would be identified as "pathological" self-blame within the incest literature, relate to my desire, no matter how futile, to perform adequately under the male gaze. Women, as well as men, judge themselves according to male norms, reinforcing the assumptions and practices of normativity.

At the same time, the "unconsciousness" with which violence is woven into discourses of masculinity in ordinary community activities leaves me

74

feeling helpless and alienated. Violence is a "normal", acceptable part of masculinity. I am back in the denial of my family of origin. I could scream and people would either not hear me or would tell me I am wrong or over-reacting. If I scream, I take up the social positioning of a stereotypical "mad woman"[20]. Authentic public acknowledgement of the horrors of childhood sexual abuse requires addressing male violence and women's marginalization as resulting from systemic power rather than individual pathology. Without this, recognition of what I have lived remains mostly confined to the "private" sphere of friends and therapy.

Because the assimilation of gendered identity is not a singular practice, possibilities exist to interrupt discourses of normativity. Judith Butler refers to gender as a "performative accomplishment" (1990:141) located in particular social and historical moments.[21] Similarly Moore (1994) identifies more than one version of masculinity or femininity. These could be brought together differently. As an example of the potential possibilities within a normative framework that appears to be monolithic, Valverde cites the development of the "green shopper," a new combination within the dichotomies of ecology and capitalism (1994). Encouraging the assimilation of disowned parts of the masculine/feminine dichotomy is the current thrust in progressive circles to shift gendered identities.

Creating new possibilities within the dichotomies of masculine and feminine can be seen in Audre Lorde's writing about her relationship with her son. She redefines strength and bravery as the capacity to love and resist. Seeing this as key for the survival of children of colour, Lorde says:

> The strongest lesson I can teach my son is the same lesson I teach my daughter: how to be who he wishes to be for himself. And the best way I can do this is to be who I am and hope that he will learn from this not how to be me, which is not possible, but how to be himself. And this means how to move to that voice inside himself, rather than to those raucous, persuasive, or threatening voices from outside, pressuring him to be what the world wants him to be. (1984:77)

In articulating the need for critical reflection about normative social discourses, Lorde asserts the possibility of a "voice inside" which can separate itself from normative discourses. While I don't disagree with this, normative discourses and individual desires live in a dynamic creative tension. Inevitably, some of who I want to be will reflect those normative discourses.

Perhaps it is in the spaces between discourses demonstrated by Valverde's "green shopper" that will give rise to alternative ways of being, thinking and doing[22].

My role as my son's mother becomes one of expanding possibilities for a masculine identity through respecting his choices, finding spaces that will challenge normativity, delighting in his developing manhood, encouraging his expressiveness, and questioning messages he receives about what masculinity requires. My power to do this requires on-going maintenance of my power in a culture which views women as sexual objects, as providers of care, as the cause of 'the problem' (Kaschak, 1992). I am as susceptible to internalizing these messages as my son. Each of us is engaged in an on-going process of negotiating our way through normative gendered discourses. On-going critical reflection to unpack what is being produced in our relationships, our assumptions, beliefs and practices, is a key beginning point. With greater awareness about myself and my relationships, the capacity for myself and others to shift normative assumptions is increased.

Chapter 5

MY BODY: SHELL OF PATRIARCHY, HOME

It isn't that we don't know. It's how do we bear what we know?
How do you bear all the ways you are hated, all the ways you
are treated with contempt, all of the ways your life is less than
it should have been? How do you feel that?
SANDRA BUTLER, 1992

One needs to study the kind of body the current society needs...
MICHEL FOUCAULT,
*Power/Knowledge Selected Interviews
and Other Writings,* 1972-1977

The process of retrieving incest memories through the therapeutic
reconnection of body with feeling has profoundly altered my relationship
to my body. For most of my life I understood this relationship through
normative standards; my body was controlled by my mind and acted as a
vehicle which carried out my wishes. When I was ill, I understood the
cause in terms of an external, like bacteria, and ignored any connection
between my illness and emotion or stress. However, recovering memory
requires taking physical sensations and feelings seriously, not rationalizing
them away. Champagne articulates this shift when she says "remembering
trauma is less about cognitive thinking than about letting go of defense
mechanisms, such as selective amnesia" (1996:110).

The physical, mental, emotional and social dislocation of recovering
traumatic memory is multi-layered, unsettling and risky. Embodied horror,
betrayal and helplessness must be grappled with and incorporated into
everyday life. The inexplicable bodily pain, the intense feelings and sleepless
nights accompanying the return of memory requires management in the
context of raising children, going to work, doing the chores. As Margaret
Randall eloquently phrased it "how do you do this work after the post

office and before class, after breakfast with a friend and after the shopping list, after protection, before the poem?" (1987: 22). Opening the body to the memory recovery process also brings unaccustomed vulnerability and a visceral awareness of daily social violences. Negotiating the world to include embodied openness and vulnerability requires time and effort and is limited at best. Articulating needs arising from memory recovery in a normative framework that will pathologize them risks marginalization. Here I trace the intersections and disjunctures between my experiences of trauma and my training in the normative discourses of the body.

Therapeutic discussion on the incest survivor's recovery process does not deal with larger questions of the implications of violation for the individual in and through normative discourses. For the most part, therapeutic discussion confines itself to understanding the memory recovery process and management of symptoms. The memory recovery process is not understood well by scientific methodologies. However, the importance of reconnecting to the body as the site where lost memory, feelings and sensation can be regained is cited throughout the therapeutic literature (Burstow, 1992; Herman, 1992; Bass & Davis, 1988).

First outlined by Janet in 1889, later by Freud, and now explored by contemporary theorists, trauma overwhelms the individual's capacity for defense and has a significant impact on the individual's embodiment:

> Traumatic events produce profound and lasting changes in physiological arousal, emotion, cognition and memory. Moreover traumatic events may sever these normally integrated functions from one another . . . Traumatic symptoms have a tendency to become disconnected from their source and to take on a life of their own. (Herman, 1992:34)

Psychoanalysis first outlined the powerful and unconscious relationship between trauma that is not consciously known and its indirect expression in everyday life. As theorized psychoanalytically, the individual seems driven by unknown forces. Once the unconscious is known and expressed, the "charge" from the past dissipates, leaving room within the individual's life for change. Champagne summarizes this work:

> If the unconscious is structured like a language (probably Lacan's most quoted concept), then aftereffects, too (since they reside in the unconscious) can be read as texts . . . Reading

aftereffects is not the simplistic project of plugging incest into a
"checklist" of symptoms but rather the complex and risky busi-
ness of giving narrative shape to symptoms and their probable
cause. (1996: 17)

With the development of feminist therapy, the survivor, not the psychia-
trist, guides the process of creating the narrative meaning of the symptoms
(Champagne, 1996).

"Forgetting" traumatic events has been explained as a way to avoid pain
and/or becoming overwhelmed. In theorizing the underlying reasons for
amnesia of childhood sexual abuse, Freyd articulates the possibility that
amnesia is related to the degree of betrayal within the traumatic event. She
outlines seven characteristics increasing the likelihood of amnesia:

1. abuse by a caretaker; 2. explicit threats demanding silence; 3.
alternative realities (abuse context different from non-abuse
context); 4. isolation during abuse; 5. young at age of abuse; 6.
alternative reality-defining statements by caregiver; 7. lack of
discussion of abuse. (1996: 140)

Freyd's survey of existing research supports her theory of the link between
betrayal and amnesia.

Other recent work in this area explores the biochemical nature of
trauma. Van der Kolk (1994) outlines the role of hormonal secretions
which reduce the impact of trauma through dulling sensation and creating
a strong "memory trace". At the same time, prolonged trauma creates
chemical change within the body resulting in an emergency hyperarousal
response to everyday events that bear a resemblance – however minimal
and (un)conscious – to the original trauma.

In addition to this work explaining the phenomena of repressed memory,
the therapeutic literature also focuses on learning and using self-care skills
to enhance safety and physical tolerance within the "recovery" process, and
to manage "symptoms" (Bass & Davis, 1988). Learning to renegotiate
destructive relationships with the body is presented in individual terms,
a project undertaken by the individual with support from close friends
or intimates.

Survivor's accounts of their bodies echo the therapeutic emphasis on
connecting to the body. Narratives begin with a growing awareness of
physical disconnection. This is followed by experiences which help the

individual gain more physical connection, and then the writing ends (Hoppen, 1994; Bass & Davis, 1988). My question in this process is what about the next day and the day after that? Most stories from therapy end with some new small triumph in regaining their body. By ending there, it seems as if the struggle is over, they have arrived. I don't want to minimize the importance of these victories. At the same time, I want to highlight that the struggle is not over tomorrow or the day after that. It will never be over. I'm aware of feeling miserable, somewhere in my body, all the time. I can move the misery around between physical and emotional pain but I can't ever seem to move beyond the misery, or if so, only for moments. It is, for me, as defining a feature as my body shape, hair colour and interests. Little has been written about the impact of on-going physical distress within the survivor's everyday life.

The therapeutic literature is also silent on how discourses of normativity will complicate the changing relationships between myself and my body. Grosz describes the body:

> By 'body' I understand a concrete, material, animate organiza-
> tion of flesh, organs, nerves and skeletal structure which are
> given unity, cohesiveness, and form through the psychical and
> social inscription of the body's surface. The body is, so to speak
> . . . a series of uncoordinated potentialities that require social
> triggering, ordering, and long term administration. (1995:104)

The body is viewed as an entity "that is manipulated, shaped, trained; which obeys, responds, becomes skilful, and increases its forces" (Foucault in Gordon, 1980:180). This training is individually-focussed and stresses economically efficient movements as well as constant coercion through normative expectations and evaluation (181). Individuals learn to perform their body in ways which reflect their social positioning.

In a culture in which rationality forms the dominant normative context, the body is fundamentally inscribed as potential and as danger through dichotomies of masculine and feminine. These dichotomies – masculinity owns the first characteristic in each pairing – include: mind/body; rational/irrational; sanity/madness; culture/nature; thought/desire. Religions such as Christianity view the body as a "fallen" state, the site of sin and deception. Bodies that cross boundaries of social convention "constitute a site of pollution and danger" (J. Butler, 1990:132). In negotiating her embrace with the realm of the body, the survivor enters dangerous terrain.

Through a biological scientific lens, knowledge about the body requires experts and has become the domain of medicine:

> We learn that the body has an elusive truth, not available to our
> own feelings, knowledge or beliefs, but rather comprehensible
> only to someone with special skills to analyze the elements of a
> symptomology which the experiencing body can't understand.
> (Berland, 1993:32)

Although the work survivors undertake is to reconnect to their bodies, within the dominant scientific framework, the body remains unknowable to all but the experts.

I begin my encounter with this "unknowable" with the dilemmas resulting from taking my experience of the feminine, the body, the irrational seriously. My exploration of these questions opens with some representations of what it is to live the process of regaining traumatic memory, to bring to the forefront the viscerality with which this process is experienced.

Remembering

When I was thirty-four I woke up one morning and didn't want to be married anymore. I didn't know why. Unlike flashes of insight I had previously ignored, this time I paid attention. At the time, my two children were preschoolers and I was studying part-time in a Masters program. One of my professors, dian Marino, was passionately and creatively alive. Her courage, strength and joy awakened me. I wanted more than the grey fog I inhabited. Now, when I look back on those years, I believe that being pregnant and giving birth twice within two years shook memories loose from their careful containment, resulting in a growing depression.

As the terrifying and painful process of questioning my marriage began, I entered marriage counselling with my husband. I continued with that therapist, learning in the process that I was skilled at talking about what I felt rather than feeling it; I preferred talk to feeling. After nearly a year, I wanted to go down to the beach and pound the sand. It was time for another way in. After about a month of seeing a bioenergetics therapist, I was sitting on the bus on my way to my appointment when I remembered myself as a child, terrified of dinosaurs on television and the pirates in "Swiss Family Robinson". When I told my therapist, she said she didn't know if I was afraid of pirates and dinosaurs but I was terrified of something. That night in bed I saw my father's shadow looming over me, felt the pain and terror of his presence.

1989

Lying in therapy for the first time floating above my body. Describing my frustration of not being able to leave my body behind without dying and not being able to live in my body. Talking about slipping into the crack in the wall beside my bed as a child.

1991

The long dark tunnel time, two years of being terrified, overwhelmed, depressed, scared. Two years of fragility, unpacking the terror, the horror. Two years of nausea accompanying physical movement. Feeling blocked. Hating it. Two years of tired, of hanging on, of intense loneliness. Two years of hoping for something better, of journeying down through numbness into grief and terror. Two years of sleeping terrified, of shadows attacking, of turning the light on. People tell me I seem better now. When they say this, I'm not sure how I seemed before. I did maintain my respectability by coping with working, going to school, caring for my children, buying a house alone during those two years.

I hate this body with its road map of memories, of terror. I would leave it if I could. I hate how it remembers and reminds me. I hate the humiliations I suffered through it.

September, 1992

I have been in massage therapy off and on for three years. The struggle to stay in my body while a stranger teaches skin, muscle and bone to stand down from its protective history has been conducted in silence.

Where I live in my body shifts from my chest to my stomach. It takes longer to leave my body when I get scared, there is more chance I can hang onto myself. Landing more in my body, I see my resistance to everything. All my energy is focused on always questioning, looking for the holes, never surrendering. Resistance constricts memory. To stop resisting is to remember, to live again the horror, the hurt, the damage locked in my body. A life sentence in this shell of patriarchy lived in the fibre of my being. I can rage at the damage but I can only accept this home, this road map of my life.

May, 1996

I feel as if I am living in the Sahara Desert and I have been asked to build a house made out of wood. There isn't a tree for hundreds of miles with which to make the boards. Any foundation would shift in the sand. I need to build a self that has a sense of itself, with limits and boundaries, destroyed long ago. Beyond caring for others there is only emptiness, a void. I could pretend and build a life, limits that look as if they are mine. For awhile I might even convince myself. I lack the energy to try anything. So I sit here amid the brokenness and wonder about acceptance of the shattered fragments that remain.

Ripped awake last night at the old time: 3:30 a.m. More memory, more terror, more visions of anal rape and something unclear. I get up to go to the bathroom. This is worse. Having to carry on was unbearable as a child. I was used as an orifice and then expected to behave as any other little girl growing up. I wanted to wet the bed as a child but I was punished. I learned to get up and carry on.

I am newly aware of the silence in which I live behind the mask. Waking up feeling nothing, counting the cracks in the ceiling as a child, counting the objects on a banner that hangs on my wall now. Knowing that somewhere in the night I was betrayed again echoed in my awakening. Not yet able to face donning the survivor's mask. Sad, hopeless and alone would be closest to what I feel in the morning and then determined to try again. Perhaps it will get better. Silence remains, imprisoning me.

June, 1996
Plagued by bouts of diarrhea as if my body is remembering its history of anal rape, enemas, violation. For years my butt has ached in/with remembering. The slightest touch feels like violation, my skin quivers in horror. Wrists and ankles wake up crossed, remembering the ropes that held them fast. Back muscles tighten, reliving the hopeless struggle to get away. My body remembers and remembers and remembers in vivid horrific detail. I live in its echoes.

Remembering is a slow, unfolding, confusing and painful process. It requires patience and tolerance for ambivalence as the wordless story emerges and takes shape. I used to hope for a single cathartic event that would "get it all out." Rather, it has turned out to be a rambling exploration that slowly clarifies before the spiral turns down into yet another layer. For a long time I quite openly wanted somewhere else to live besides in my body.

Negotiating The "Polluted" Body

There is an on-going edge to the memory retrieval process of living in a body that has participated – however unwillingly – in activities that lie outside of what we are told are the norms of social convention. (A definition that is ironic, given the "normalcy" of violation in the lives of many women and children.) These experiences have left me with a visceral experience of feeling "polluted", grappling to establish a sense of bodily integrity. I experience enormous shame about my bodily responses during the violation, how my sexuality may have been shaped through the abuse. Emotional and physical needs for comfort and connection, as well as feelings of vulnerability, also raise shame. While feminist therapy creates new discourses through which women can understand their symptoms, affirm their need for relationship, and place appropriate responsibility on abusers, I continue to feel the impact of normative discourses. This sense of difference, of knowledge and experience outside social norms, contributes to my alienation, the watcher who looks on and does not participate.

This sense of inhabiting a "polluted" body also reflects the historical legacy of the eugenics movement, with its idea of "tainted" genetic inheritances (Walkerdine, 1984). I sometimes feel as if I am replicating my parents. Many of my bodily changes resemble my father. The protruding veins below the skin on my hands, the strong but tiny ankle bones and wrists of a Welsh coal-mining heritage; his chronic indigestion. Sometimes I feel haunted again by his presence and fear that I am becoming him. In the struggle to use trifocals, having at last succumbed to wearing glasses, I feel like my mother wearing her bifocals. My head tilts like a bird in search of the spot through which I can see clearly. I hesitate, as she did, before descending a flight of stairs. Sometimes I'm amused, often I am not. It requires discipline to maintain the reality of my inheritance, memories of my parents and my separate existence. Even though I understand my incest experiences predominantly through feminist therapeutic discourses, I continue to viscerally experience the effects of normative discourses which judge my morality and genetic inheritance.

Negotiating the Rational-Irrational Dichotomy

The process of uncovering and affirming repressed traumatic memory fundamentally inverts the normative dominance of rationality. What may be seen as a survivor's struggle with self-blame, may also be understood as a difficulty in developing a normative and socially-acceptable sense of self, when normative frameworks locate memory retrieval as irrational or mad. This boundary, between the rational and the irrational, may be negotiated in a multitude of ways.

Initially, I found it difficult to temporarily silence my rational internal editor who had protected my story and my "public" presentation for many years. The process of recovering memory lands the survivor squarely within the realm of the irrational, the world of madness, a world traditionally controlled by men. According to Phyllis Chesler, a woman is defined as mad "when she acts out her thoughts and feelings with her body ... without any group support or consensus" (1972:89). When I questioned the "truth" of what my body was experiencing, my therapist told me my choice was either follow the process through or believe I was mad. The world of the mad is one of social marginalization and regulation through hospitalization and drugs. Partly due to my race and class privilege, I have remained directly untouched by this medicalization of my madness. Indirectly, the potential dangers of being pathologized led me, until now, to live this process in silence with all but a trusted few.

Despite my avoidance of medical intervention, the world of the mad continued to haunt me. For many years, I feared a return of memory that would push me over the defined edge of rationality, to where I would no longer be able to carry out my daily routine. The recent realization my embodiment is already handling all my rage, grief and shame has helped. Therapy is a process of house-cleaning; reorganizing the cupboards, so to speak. When I am remembering, I'm not sure I can handle the intensity of emotion. What I have not recognized is that I am already handling it. This increases my certainty that having survived it once and carried on, I can probably survive it again. I am not in danger of completely losing control and going "crazy", I have already dealt with this once. The choice is not about whether to remember, but about how.

The scientific focus on eradicating symptoms has also been an underlying theme throughout my therapeutic process. I have openly longed for my therapist to take away the pain; later for me to find the "magic" solution. Where is the salve that will cure me? If I move to the country, if I get angry, if I eat right will that take away the pain? I am a broken record of scientific normative discourse in search of a single solution.

Bringing Language to the Irrational

If the discourses of scientific pathology form one boundary of the rational-irrational dichotomy the survivor must negotiate, then language forms another. Part of the encoding of memory into rationality depends on bringing language to the traumatic experience in an embodied state. Van der Kolk (1994) refers to the "speechless terror" of the survivor while Chandler (1990) describes the survivor's "wordless, nameless grieving state". Laub outlines this struggle to express trauma in language when he says:

There are never enough words or the right words, there is never enough time or the right time, and never enough listening or the right listening to articulate a story that cannot fully be captured in thought, memory and speech. (1995: 63)

While bringing language to the experience of trauma is part of integrating memory, the nature of language means some of the experience is inevitably left behind. In his discussion of the young child learning language, Stern outlines the limits of language:

> ... language is a double-edged sword. It also makes some parts of our experience less shareable with ourselves and with others. It drives a wedge between two simultaneous forms of experience: as it is lived and as it is verbally represented ... Language, then, causes a split in the experience of the self. (1985:162)

Distance is created between the embodied experience and its expression in language. The relationship between lived experience and expression in language is made more complex when Stern talks of language's role in encoding "official or socialized world knowledge" (1985:178). Experience may by excluded from expression in language or it may be framed in particular ways. For me, there was always this struggle about what I would leave behind by speaking and how what I would say could be most accurately framed in language. My reluctance to speak about what I was experiencing was both terror in breaking silence and the difficulty of bringing language accurately to the child's experience. Although the therapeutic literature describes difficulties breaking silence, there is little discussion of this struggle with language.

Moving carefully through the process of remembering, and not superimposing explanations on the memories, is critical for the survivor to emerge with language that fits (Burstow, 1992). I have experienced this phenomenon when remembering an intense sensation. For a while I wondered if I had given birth to a baby when I was a young person, because I had the extraordinary desire to bear down, full of terror. Sifting and sorting through the sensations I experienced with the knowledge I have, I arrived at the explanation of enduring enemas; this fits with what I know of my family and childhood. Staying open to possibilities, without imposing explanations through language, is crucial if I want to bring my memories home, to become part of who I am rather than remain unknown and fragmented. Otherwise, disownment of my memories will continue in the name of a particular theory or explanation. If there is any value to the position of False Memory Syndrome in doubting the veracity of repressed memory, it is in raising the question of what explanations are being super-imposed by whom.

The lack of language in the traumatic experiences of a tiny child adds to the sense of the irrationality in memory retrieval. The fantastical quality of remembering, the eeriness, the larger-than-life horror reflects how a child experiences abuse. Everything in the world looks big from the perspective of a small child. There is a foreshortening quality to remembering that reflects the child's vision. The intensity of sensation and emotion, unmediated by language, is what a baby experiences as a memory storage system. This fantastical quality of reentering a traumatized child's world makes it difficult to accept memories returning into a social context where rationality dominates.

Reintegrating the Irrational

Perhaps because of the fantastical quality of memory retrieval, I worked for a long time to find a rational narrative which would explain my embodied memories. Because returning memory appears in segments and fragments, dribs and drabs, locating a narrative was a formidable task. I wanted the story to bring a rational explanation to what I was feeling, to reduce the sense of being "mad". As more of me remembers through simultaneously being less numb and less terrified, my desire for a coherent narrative is reduced. Having survived "madness" I am less invested in maintaining the boundaries between the rational and the "mad", between explanation and feelings[23].

The integration of traumatic memory into other parts of my life has been a slow process. I lived the rational and irrational as parallel experiences. Looking back to my first time in therapy, when I allowed myself to experience floating above my body, disappearing into a crack in the wall, my profile fit the "classic" incest framework survivors have built through understanding their processes. At the time, I understood it just as a very weird experience. As my tolerance and interest grew, so too did my knowledge. Writing has provided a clearer sense of my process. Taking in the implications of the therapeutic work slowly, over time, has been important in allowing me to claim incest as an accurate portrait of my experience, based on sifting and sorting, not on an imposed explanation.

Because memory is stored in the body, in a sense, I haven't remembered anything that I wasn't already aware of in some way. This awareness may be vague; it may live as well-ingrained habits of captivity designed to keep terror and rage at bay. Or it may have more definition. Examples of this in my life include knowing how much I disliked my father for as long as I can remember, how unhappy I felt below the surface of the mask. What becomes possible to know, however, changes; as well as what it is possible to name and state individually and socially (Butler, 1992).

Reintegrating retrieved memory also begins to shift dichotomous patterns and decisions established long ago. There is a black and white, either/or quality to the experience of my traumatized child and decisions she made. Remembering always takes me into a life and death struggle. As I work in the present to undo some of the legacies of the past, I see my child's construction of the world, her decisions. For example, if I sense someone isn't likely to listen to me, I remain masked and do not speak at all about what I experience or need. I withdraw from people in disagreement, in anger or hurt, almost before my emotions register. Over time, sudden withdrawal has become a signpost to consider whether a more complex response is possible.

How I live in my body has also shifted through the reintegration process. One of the more elusive costs from my point of view is the loss of my capacity to transcend the body through the close similarity between trance-like states and dissociation (Culbertson, 1995). Coming to live in my body means abandoning transcendence, a return to the mundaneness of earth after flying through the universe. It means taking the world seriously as is, rather than focussing on its transformative potential. This seems a pedestrian and painful undertaking. Losing transcendence is part of my grief. But transcendence was also part of my alienation, my sense of being dismissed as idealistic or ignored.

With this cost comes a growing sense of the interconnectedness of life forms. As a child, while outdoors, I sensed a connectedness to the universe that felt like an acknowledged call for help. For several years after I began to regain my lost stories, all this connection was lost. It was almost as if the answer to my call for help was "stop depending on me, grow up". I have regained moments of knowing I am held within the universe, part of something larger. Now, I have a growing awareness of connectedness, as if my life is part of but not the same as, all other life forms. I am individual and share universality in the same breath. Throughout this process I have been struck by the tenacity to which I have held onto life, even when death seemed to promise relief. I have learned the power with which life calls to us and holds us. If life seems remotely possible, then it is life I will choose.

Negotiating the Irrational Body in the World

Integration of repressed memory and realignment of past patterns within the present shift how the survivor lives within the world. Because normative discourses which dichotomize mind and body, rational and irrational, thought and feeling, well and ill have not changed, the survivor living in a traumatized body is constantly negotiating these dichotomies. The following journal entries trace some of the dilemmas underlying this process.

Because of chronic tiredness, sore throats and indigestion, I began to see a naturopath. Her questions about thirst, body temperature, food cravings, fears and emotions wove a sense of the interconnectedness between my habits, my feelings and my body. She worked on strengthening my immune system, predominantly through diet. After about a year I decided to try a two week cleansing diet. This placed me on a collision course with normative discourses surrounding the body.

June 13, 1993
It is day four of the diet. I should be feeling better and I'm not. My body is not doing what other people's bodies do. I am on a slippery slide out of control, back into the incest. Any shift away from the "safety" of my mother's routine leaves me alone, hopeless and beaten once again.

June 15, 1993
I feel slowed down today. I'm noticing flowers and can't be bothered to run for the subway.

June 16, 1993
I don't feel as if I have any skin today. I feel very vulnerable. I don't know how to live in the workplace feeling vulnerable. I want caffeine and sugar to rev me up and away from feeling abandoned, despairing, violated. I feel nourished on this diet and my digestion is better. My skin crawls with desire for comfort food.

August 26, 1993
I'm still struggling around food, tired of juggling what the kids will eat with what I should eat. At the same time I feel better. I've lost weight, have lots of energy and feel less ashamed of my body. When I "cheat" I don't enjoy it as much as I had anticipated.

Eating requires so much planning. It is very difficult to grab something when I am out. I feel surrounded by a culture in which the commodification of food is completely divorced from nourishment. I feel as if I am swimming against a tidal wave of caffeine, sugar, wheat and grease. No one strolls down to a local parlour to enjoy a raw carrot or a piece of fruit. Desire and pleasure are divorced from health.

In the workplace the needs of my body are secondary to the structure of the job. After five hours on the telephone problem-solving with people, I need to stretch, take a walk, shift gears physically, mentally and emotionally. Making soup or doing laundry would rebalance me. There are several more hours to go. I am required to stay. I can't find much flexibility to bring some needed relief. As I plug in the kettle to make herbal tea, other women are pouring coffee or eating chocolate.

Meetings go on past the point of my endurance because it is "cost-efficient" in terms of travel. I am paid to meet the demands of the organization and ignore my own. I feel as if my efforts to live in my body are acts of resistance in a culture designed to numb its citizens. In a committee meeting discussing an up-coming weekend of training, one powerful volunteer states that if you are being paid to attend you should be willing to work from six a.m. to midnight. These high expectations and long hours are common in non-profit "caring" organizations as well as other parts of the working world. I have a clear sense of what this costs me in terms of fatigue, and being unable to hold my ground.

May, 1996
Back on the cleansing diet. Cravings for caffeine and sugar are gone. I feel slowed down from my usual driven-ness. I'm very much in the moment. I loved seeing all the people on the subway today, walking home in the soft spring evening. I am so open to what is around me. This is very unlike where I usually live in which my body is an instrument of accomplishment driven towards its goals. Emotionally I am unprotected, vulnerable. There is energy here for the next task as it presents itself. It is energy of response rather than accomplishment.

I have never felt so alive as I do right now. Everything around me has come alive overnight, as spring burst late over Toronto. My life resonates with the life around me. Whatever I am doing is wonderful, simply because I am alive in a world that is full of life.

I feel like a piece of paper towelling absorbing the energy of those around me. I can not live continually with people for very long before I am confused as to where I end and they begin. Their reactions, feelings become absorbed into me. For all that I can process what is mine, what is not mine in all of this, and clear myself out, the fact that I absorb as easily as I breathe remains. Sometimes I think there is tremendous power in my capacity to enter in so completely.

An old friend tells me I don't seem as angry as I used to. I can't seem to conjure up the same levels of self-blame anymore. I seem more able to tolerate complexity in myself and in the world.

February 12, 1997
For some months now I have been taking a substantial amount of medication to treat candida. Occasionally I worry about what the medication may be doing to my body's balance. Rather than feeling sick, mostly I feel as if my body is recovering and that I can tolerate its process. I have not had this much energy since I was twenty-five. In the evening I feel naturally tired but not exhausted or hyper. I look forward to the day, not as physically depressed somehow. The diet restrictions anger me. I bargain with myself to do as much as will make me well, rather than make a more long term dietary change. If I seek quick access to comfort food in the context of a busy life, I am automatically "off" the diet. I find the constant need to plan and prepare food unbearable.

July 7, 1997
My body seems to be reacting to the intense work of articulating the analysis of this work. My ears are itchy, red, inflamed with eczema which is spreading to my eyelids. Fungus is beginning to grow again. I can see my body reacting to my breaking of silence. I have patiently applied the cream that will heal but not suppress the symptoms. I seem to be hitting a wall here. I want medicine that will take the symptoms away. My patience with itching and a boring diet is at an end.

In the writing process I have lost any clarity I fleetingly possess with respect to my body. I feel as miserable in my body now as I did as a child with vague complaints and nothing really wrong. I feel awash in my life, drifting, unclear how to care for myself, wishing someone would cook and shove it under my nose, leaving me free to write.

August, 1997
I'm wondering if I know anything at all about living in my body. Through blood tests, the doctor identified indicators of what she calls pre-cancerous levels of stress. Three weeks off is her recommendation. At this point I would not know what to do with a holiday. I chuckle at how she identifies the causes of stress as external to the individual. Trauma doesn't seem to take time off. I have relied on my stamina to maintain my life. Now it appears to be leaving me.

As I talk to others about how they managed the writing process, I am aware of my driven-ness, the quality I associated most with my father. At the moment the best I seem to be able to do is to learn to take my foot off the gas. The deeper sources of stress learned in the past feel much more difficult to shift. Every risk is accompanied by my terror of being wrong and being punished. My mother's coldness towards my physical comfort, my abuse, betrayal and rage live on in my driven-ness. My mind, not my body, brings pleasure.

Normative Expectations and A Traumatized Body

Feeling embodied leaves me vulnerable, open to my feelings, to others, to stimulation from my surroundings, as well as past memory. At the same time, normative control of the mind over the body creates performative standards I can only meet by numbing out. These include long hours, repetitive work and multiple demands on my time and energy. Denial and minimization help individuals cope with this "insidious trauma" of capitalist oppression (Root in Brown, 1995). Interestingly enough, readily available food – caffeine, sugar and fat – rev the body to meet these performative demands and are culturally associated with comfort in North America.

I feel caught between the demands of the world and the embodiment I am learning. My struggle to create a discursive space which will acknowledge and support integrating these dichotomies is individualized and lacking in tangible models. When my stress levels are described as pre-cancerous, I wonder: how out of touch am I really? I pose this question as someone who rarely drinks or smokes and who does not do drugs. As a survivor, where do I fall with respect to numbness within the general population?

Because the conditions of insidious trauma resonate with those of earlier trauma, I am driven to perform or endure in an effort to ensure some safety and ward off further punishment (Burstow, 1992). Each sunrise defines the tasks to be done and each sunset measures my success or sloth, my worthiness or worthlessness. When I can no longer perform, I collapse into an inert ball of pain, terrified of my vulnerability and helpless to act on my own behalf. Maintaining embodiment is not just a question of learning to balance time and activities. It requires the capacity to hold mind, body and feelings in each particular moment, to learn to be with some sense of certainty and safety. This is destroyed by traumatic oppression.

What makes full embodiment so elusive is my inability to define what I need in a normative dichotomy of health or illness. Sometimes, after a sleepless night full of memory, or in periods of prolonged depression, the best thing I can do is force myself back into the present by going to work.

However, the demands of the workplace may outstrip my capacity to meet them, leaving me exhausted and without a viable explanation. It is often easier to stay in a driven mode rather than try to negotiate the morass of what my mind-body-feelings might require. Knowing that if I am unable to perform according to normative standards I can be marginalized – informally, through a reputation for "unreliability", or formally through a diagnosed illness – also contributes to my driven-ness (Berland, 1993). I am left caught between normative standards of performance and the ambiguous symptoms of a traumatized body.

Never Measuring Up - Reverberations and Competence

Average physical competence for adults includes such activities as riding a bike, ice skating, negotiating slippery surfaces easily, moving furniture, responding quickly to perceived danger. As a survivor I am constantly negotiating these average expectations in a body that cannot perform, cannot be counted on. I become anxious in situations where I know what is regarded as normal will be insurmountable. Knowing that I may freeze in response to danger makes me careful in selecting the activities I undertake. I monitor where, with whom, and how I will spend time, stunting my sense of adventure and risk-taking.

Two short anecdotes reveal the everyday nature of my encounters with normative standards defining what I should be able to do, but am not.

On vacation in Haliburton, Ontario in August 1992, there is a fairly steep path from the cottage down to the water full of rocks, tree roots, bumps. The children, and a friend visiting for a few days, skip down unconcerned. I pick my way, feeling the exhaustion of the past year and the usual humiliation of being off city cement. When I am this tired, my fear is greater.

I am last in the lake, disliking the cold, uncomfortable with the bouncing of the children on and off the raft, feeling like a taut, fragile piece of glass, terrified I will panic in their unpredictability. I long to play with them, to swim across the lake with them. I long to support their growing certainty in their bodies with more than praise, as my friend can and does.

I try learning to drive a gearshift. I have to back the car up a steep slope. I freeze, each time, stalling the car, terrified of what feels like braking the car to let the clutch out as I give it gas. This is not safe. My feet do not trust changing their driving habits. I sit in defeat, humiliated once again.

Years later, in the winter of 1997, I arrive in the small town of Bracebridge, Ontario with a volunteer to meet with the board of directors of one of our local agencies. A steep icy hill runs from the parking lot to the front door of the building. Knowing the potential for humiliation, I say to the volunteer, "I don't do ice, let's try going in the back." She looks at me strangely, surprised, and makes a reference to the others about my difficulty during a general discussion of the icy conditions.

It is the evaluative nature of normative standards which creates the threat within these brief narratives. There is the potential for judgement in pathological or incompetent terms by my friend, my children, my colleague, which will shape what they ask me to (not) do and what they think of me. Although nothing may be said, the strength of normative evaluative standards shapes what others think of me and what I think of myself. In the present these conditions reverberate with past abuse, where the dangers of being vulnerable or incompetent in managing the abuse were indeed high. The reverberation between evaluative conditions in the present and past trauma leaves me continually struggling with shame, self-blame and an intense sense of embodied pathology. This is as much about the conditions of the present as it is about the past.

While my physical incompetence continues to haunt me and leave me vulnerable, how I perform my presentation of my body in the world reveals the intersection of my incest history with my social locations of race, class, gender and sexual orientation.

Invisibility and Comfort

When I think back, presentation of my body has been lodged in invisibility and comfort. Bulky clothing protected me from the outside world. Comfort, as well as colour, not fashion or sex appeal, were the guiding threads from which I chose. High heels, nylons, skirts, make-up are worn as little as possible. Looking a little bit different was much more important that looking "nice" or "like a girl". Dressing to attract sexual attention remains incomprehensible. What strikes me in any discussion regarding my body is the impossibility of neutrality. My body is never allowed to be just a body.

More recently, I'm grateful for all the ways in which my relationship with my body is peaceful and enjoyable. Most of it is private pleasure in my sense of material existence, how my body feels as I sit quietly or move through the world, the on-going pleasure in bodily functions, of applying lotion to skin with muscle and bone, of water cascading on skin and hair, the hollow, jiggling sound of a rounded stomach played like a drum. These pleasures are private, rarely discussed. The private is also not always pleasurable. Like other women I can evaluate my best features and those which are inadequate, too large or too small in my view (Kaschak, 1992).

Living in my body in the world feels like a bombardment of messages in which I am at risk as an object of desire or a source of derision. The messages vary from the slightly raised eyebrows of my teenaged daughter as she enters the bathroom during the completion of my morning routine, to my desire to always be covered in the presence of my teenaged son. I know that I, too, raise eyebrows or purse lips in judgement at other bodies. Decisions I make at work regarding who is the "best" representative for the organization in different situations depends partly on their bodily presentation. Those with power also make similar decisions about me.

I feel surrounded by media images of women's bodies selling entrance to a life of success, ease and comfort. This objectification bombards me with reminders of how I am still at risk, how I am viewed through a narrow lens in which my female body is all that is important about me (Kaschak,1992; Burstow,1992).

Out in the world I am constantly faced with issues of bodily presentation. How to present my material self as a mother (who is not embarrassing), a lesbian (who is cool), a worker juggling a multitude of roles, requiring gradations of material presentation from friendly to official, across urban and rural settings. In addition to this, I am faced with cultural representations of the female body from advertisements, art and film.

Most of the time my response is negation, not of pleasure in achieving a particular "look". I want to look clean, healthy and tidy, but not like an athlete or Pollyanna. I want to look attractive but not attract unwanted sexual attention. I want to look like a lesbian but not so extreme that I risk rejection or danger in small rural communities. I want to look like a professional but not so professional that I become unapproachable, intimidating. My desire for comfort outweighs all the rest. I don't want to bother with this negotiation.

The simple question of what to wear in the morning reveals the complexity of how traumatic experience continues to thrive in my life. On the one hand, my heightened awareness of the need for social acceptability, my desire to avoid judgement and establish safety, leaves me aiming for the middle of the requirements of the social discourses in and through which I live my life. In this way, I demonstrate my capacity to negotiate the "insidious trauma" of being perceived as a sexual object (Kaschak, 1992).

On the other hand, how I dress feels like an on-going rebellious debate with the dictates of my father (the tailor), my mother (the lady) and normative expectations of white, middle-class, professional women. In this place, I am guided by what I can get away with to enhance my comfort and help me appear as casual as possible. There is an alienated refusal in this to personify my body as an object of male desire or that of a white, middle-class, professional. What I seem to embrace is resistance to the dictates of any normative discourse whether it be for mothers, lesbians, or white, middle-class professionals. This leaves me in an on-going state of unease regarding possible censure. While I may be uneasy, I am also not instantly identified as "other". The whiteness of my skin assures my inclusion, as does my middle-class professionalism. This social privilege mediates against the terror of childhood trauma and creates some possibility for me to resist normative performative discourses.

Beyond Fragmentation

Reconnecting my body and feelings leaves me with a heightened awareness of the depth of social inscriptions of the body. In my efforts to regain traumatic memory, to integrate body, mind and feeling, and to negotiate my way through the world, I am constantly encountering the edges of what is possible in normative discourses. These demands replay the experience of captivity and contribute to my sense of fragmentation. While fragmentation is conceptualized as a defensive response to trauma, it is also reinforced through normative discourses. Flax outlines this when she writes:

> The existence of asymmetrical gender relations, the ways in which the asymmetries of race encourage splitting off (and disavowal) of parts of the self (Palmer; Smith), the use of homophobia to enforce repression of sexuality and relations with others all converge to structure the "inner" world . . . Consideration of the absence, repression and mutilation of this autonomous self pushes us "outside" to become agents who can confront aggressively "civilization and its discontents". (1987:105)

Flax reconceptualizes this fragmentation of race, class and gender relations as it is currently lived into an autonomous self which would re-weave the fragments to include competition, ambition, the use of logic, the expression of feelings and caring, the ability to be alone, the desire of a sexual self, the limits of a rational one, connections to others that are neither fused nor domineering. While this holistic self cannot be achieved within the current normative context, understanding social investments in maintaining fragmentation reassures me that some of my difficulties in reconnecting body, mind and feeling relate to normative discourses. The process of learning to live in my body provides a valuable tool in uncovering how oppression is lived everyday, and brings hope that this process may uncover new possibilities in being and remaining alive rather than numb.

Chapter 6

A FRAGILE POWER

If I could live without relationships, I would choose to. There has been so much hurt, betrayal and confusion. I have not been able to manage living completely alone.

All that we have in relationships is our on-going willingness to stay in connection, to live out our affection, to be present to another person's struggles, perceptions and being as well as our own, knowing that these relationships will ultimately end. This takes courage and the affirmation of love, a fragile power.

As an incest survivor, I experience relationships as sites of longing for connection and fear of betrayal. The memory and teachings of incest live on, not only in my body, but in my approach to, and expectations of, relationships. The therapeutic literature on incest survivors focusses on how survivors' behaviour deviates from normative relational expectations through unpredictability and inconsistency. Describing how survivors behave in relationships, Herman says:

> The survivor oscillates between intense attachment and terrified withdrawal. She may cling desperately to a person whom she perceives as a rescuer, flee suddenly from a person she suspects to be a perpetrator or an accomplice, show great loyalty and devotion to a person she perceives as an ally, and heap wrath and scorn on a person who appears a complacent bystander. The roles she assigns to others may change suddenly, as the result of small lapses or disappointments . . . Over time, as most people fail the survivor's exacting tests of trustworthiness, she tends to withdraw from relationships. The isolation of the survivor thus persists even after she is free. (1992: 93)

A more complex understanding of the survivor's experience in relationship can be seen by analyzing how domination is embedded within normative relational standards. Incest is only one relational site among many in which hierarchies of power and privilege are established, taught and maintained. This hierarchy has established a male subject who attains his desire through a feminine object who responds to his desire (Benjamin, 1988). Within this duality, women "lose" their agency as desiring subjects and men "lose" their capacity for nurturance, vulnerability and dependence. Because this pattern of domination underlies normative relationships, the survivor is continually encountering experiences which resonate with her history of incest.

The survivor's response to this normative pattern may be to employ the survival mechanisms of the past by focussing her desires and actions on the interests of those with power. Champagne refers to this as "incested agency" (1996: 165). Through recognition of and identification with the subject position, the survivor hopes for the attainment of her desire (Benjamin 1988). Because subject-object relations are sites of betrayal, the survivor's task becomes learning to resist relationships of domination and to engage within subject-subject relational patterns which have the potential to transform the normativity of domination.

This discussion begins by tracing the normative relational patterns and the lessons in power and privilege they teach; it ends with possibilities for reconceptualizing desire based on subject-subject positioning.

The Normative Standard: Heterosexual Monogamy

> However we choose to identify ourselves, however we find
> ourselves labelled, it [the lie of compulsory female heterosexuality]
> flickers across and distorts our lives.
> ADRIENNE RICH,
> "Compulsory Heterosexuality and Lesbian Existence"
> in Blood, Bread and Poetry

I have a home but the desire for an "ideal" home, for a life of security, beauty and mutual recognition remains intense, as does my terror of dependence, of boredom and of my agency.

I am curious about this desire, how it lies at the feet of some unknown person, of what we would create together. In spite of thirteen years of living up close to another person in marriage, my longing for an "ideal" life with a

*partner remains. My eye rolling cynicism speaks to the depth of hurt and
need, as well as the struggle to trust myself within close relationships.*

Heterosexual monogamy as the dominant site of intimacy regulates all our
relationships, not just those of a sexual nature. How intimacy and desire are
experienced and understood, how obligation is defined, and how priorities
are established are shaped by the lens of heterosexual normativity. The
relationship with one's partner as the site of greatest intimacy, desire and
obligation, presides over other relationships. Denial of parts of the self, as
well as physical and emotional numbness, may be required to sustain the
long term presence of another person living in close everyday proximity.

> *I want longevity, consistency, security, genuine affection and caring. The
> cost of this desire has been domination, deadening, and dishonesty.
> What begins in hope may end in captivity and despair. I fear uncer-
> tainty and insecurity.*

Feminists have written extensively about heterosexual monogamy as a site
of gender domination in which women and children are subordinate to
the power and privilege of men. Women's role is one of nurturing men and
children within the family. Violence against women and children is common
within heterosexual marriage. This gendered dichotomy, which positions
females as objects of desire and creates entitlement of men's desire within
families, leaves female children at risk of childhood sexual abuse (Jacobs,
1994; Kaschak, 1992).

Within this stratified system of power and privilege, incest survivors receive
powerful lessons in normative relations. Kadi makes this link when she says:

> Child sexual abuse teaches children about social/cultural hierar-
> chies in ways that ensure we'll remember the gist of it (if not the
> details). Stamping information on bodies and imprinting it into
> body memory guarantees a high retention rate. This information
> necessarily covers more than sexism, since sexism isn't the sole
> source of oppression; racism, classism, ableism, and the systematic
> oppression of children also figure into these lessons. (1996: 74)

Survivors learn to focus on valuing, anticipating and meeting the needs
and interests of those with power and privilege (Jacobs, 1994; Champage,
1996). Within this education into normative relations of domination, I can

99

trace three particular lessons from my incest experiences that explicate relations of domination.

Normative Lessons From Captivity
1. Obey My Version of Reality

Lying watching scared, knowing that struggling, yelling, running and hiding are pointless. Hoping if I'm very good, it won't hurt this time.

Her hands run over my body, arousing my genitals. The enema water rushes into me, searing, hot, nauseating, sexual, overwhelming, let me die.

Being held down and raped seems cleaner than this frozen-in-the-headlights obedience, this emotional blackmail that dictates I cooperate and submit to being sexually aroused and then purged. I burn with rage and my own impotence in the face of this "affection", her view that her actions are for my own good.

I am left with an ingrained obedient response to demands placed on me within a relationship, whether it be in friendship, a sexual "coupled" relationship, or a professional "work" connection. Relationships seem governed by unequal power in which connection with another person and denial of myself are unequivocally linked. Except in isolation, trust in being all of myself feels impossible. I vacillate in relationship between obedience and rebellion in "incested agency", wanting to experience more of myself than is possible. The person I am in relationship with seems focused on maintaining their dominance, their certainty. While my rebellion contains the volatility that Herman deplores, it also contains the potential to move out of this dynamic of domination.

There is a familiar pattern in this on-going dynamic. In the hope of winning an affectionate heart, a warm fire to sit by, I will abandon parts of myself for a while, ignoring their demands as mine were ignored by my abusers. Rather than speak up, negotiate and choose, I finally erupt, the unheeded parts of myself tiring of their alienation. By then the relationship is established on false premises, on some but not all my needs, making trust and negotiation difficult, particularly in the complexity of another person's history, longing and needs.

The flip side of this obedience to the demands of another is my rebellion at imposed limits and refusal to fully open my heart, never risking my shell of protection against the betrayal, the final death of hope. My watcher and critic continue to look out for me. Interwoven in this withholding is my fear of another's desire, which burns down deep, beyond where I can hold onto it from the present.

Sometimes my rebellion results in a silent retreat out of relationship. Other times, it results in a power struggle. When my disobedience erupts, demands made of me seem "reasonable" by normative standards. My lack of cooperation is unthinkable. In my confusion, it takes a long time for me to articulate how I am being asked to live in someone else's conception of relationship, how my needs and perspectives are refused, how I remain unseen. Rather than affirm my silencing, confront someone's actions and refuse to comply, I rage in ambivalence, trying to convince the "other", hoping to be seen, and terrified that once again, I am feeling and/or being erased. Those who have been caught in this cycle with me might speak of how they have felt erased, unseen by me.

While this power struggle breaks the silence of my childhood, it remains caught in a subject-object relational dynamic in which each person requires the other to adopt their perspective. An alternative may be to tolerate complexity, uncertainty; to navigate through and sustain connection within multiple perspectives. Negotiation – not seduction – and tolerance of fear are skills needed to traverse this unknown ground.

2. Meet Other's Needs; Don't Delineate Your Own

Long ago I buried my need for respect for my body, for trust in others, for trust in myself. Living in domination, in the cracks and crevasses of trust and respect, requires discipline to wall off and contain my need, longing and desire.

In normative relations of desire based on subject-object, the needs of the subject are legitimated over those of the object. For incest survivors, this lesson in the erasure of their needs comes early and is reinforced by the normative standard of heterosexual monogamy in which women are the caretakers of men and children.

How much have I been rewarded for calibrating my needs to others, for caretaking, for niceness? If I listened to others, if I took care of them, then I could be with them. I survive on the glow of my caring for others. It is a habit community, work, family and marriage reward as an ideal of femininity. If the underbelly of that care is terror of being alone, of disowned need, then it is dependence and resentment that is created, not love. Escaping the trap of caretaking means exploring my aloneness, my terror, my need, to discover what is satisfying. I want to be a subject in relationship with other subjects, not a provider of care living on crumbs of affection.

In a normative framework in which women are objects, how does feminine desire constitute and legitimate itself in everyday life? Describing Irigaray's conception of male sexuality as the known and female sexuality as the unknown, Grosz says:

> Female sexuality, lesbian desire, is that which eludes and escapes, that which functions as an excess, a reminder uncontained by and unrepresentable within the terms provided by a sexuality that takes it as straightforwardly being what it is. (1995: 222)

What could be understood, in individualistic therapeutic terms, as the survivor's struggle to reincorporate desire into her identities, also reflects her position as female with her desire positioned as the unknown within the assumptions and practices of normativity. Interestingly enough, although what I experience is need, the literature focusses its discussion on desire. I wonder if need can be understood as desire experienced from the subordinated position of an object?

Feb. 12, 1997
How subtle the erasures of self are: withdrawal rather than speech, compromise, rationalize, facilitate for others. How deep is my hatred of my need, my longing for connection. My capacity to adjust silently to the conditions of my life frightens me. I get glimmers of the depth of my self-hate, the sword it holds in judgment over my everyday actions not to be an imposition, not to let the past explode all over the present, not to expose who and what I am, not to deserve the life I want.

August, 1997
Without need there is no connectedness, no certainty of my importance to someone else or their's to me.

With love comes hope and my need, longing and desire, as well as the embodied memories of betrayal, crack open. I am unprepared when the walls barricading need, longing and desire come down, terrified of being laughed at, ignored or dismissed.

Within these journal entries the legacies of incest are visible. There is the terror of breaking out of the automatic adjustments to others, the silence which guarantees "safety" (however false this may be), and the self-hate which protects the child from the full impact of the knowledge that his or her caretakers are abusive. Thinking that one is bad offers some possibility in an environment of broken trust and denial (Miller, 1990). Without the child's dependence and vulnerability, the need for these survival mechanisms would not be as crucial. As an independent adult, the survivor remains caught in this same struggle. Without awareness of need and vulnerability, the relational connection is limited.

What compounds this problem are normative gendered frameworks in which need is presented as weakness and dependence, characteristic of subordinated femininity. Being vulnerable in relationship, I am identified with this position. As a child, I learned well the price of being in this position. At the same time, my survival as a child depended on my strength to maintain a mask and not collapse within crazy-making dynamics. I associate safety with the numb independence and autonomy associated with masculinity. I struggle towards a representation of power which affirms, rather than degrades, vulnerability and need.

Within the normative framework, any possibility for meeting my needs and desires requires me to engage the subject-object power dynamic which echoes my incest history. Allowing the presence of need and desire, with choice about whether or not to engage with someone else, is not part of the normative power dichotomy. The possibility of reconceptualizing desire can be seen in Champagne's reading of Lacan, when she says:

> Desire is an unconscious state of waiting and withholding, not a conscious wish for satiation, fulfilment, completion, or closure. To fulfil a desire is to render it either pleasure or horror . . . Desire constitutes a subject and thus should not be acted on, acted out, or made material; it just need be. (1996: 144 & 145)

The capacity to hold desire within the self, as fundamental to the experience of the self, begins to move away from a subject-object power relation of domination. How this is lived in relation to others remains a source of confusion to me.

When I am seen, loved, and someone is honest with me, I am plunged into so much pain I am left reeling. I want warmth, comfort, quiet, solitude. The thought of being pushed away opens my chest, bringing raw and ancient grief.

I have lived the discipline of containing the needs of my child self, knowing that the time to have those needs met is long past. Being driven by past needs in relationship with others will derail connectedness. I need to know I can withstand the echoes and reverberations of horror, the needs of others and hold my life in the present to reach out for moments of love and connection. I need to make peace with what feels like my bottomless need. Learning I can grieve what was never met brings hope that something could grow beyond this sterility.

Because masculinity, with its ideals of a unified, controlled, independent self, acts as the baseline of maturity, the eruption of need and raw hurt from the past can only be understood by myself and others as "abnormality". Therefore, witnessing the aftermath of trauma is confined to and legitimated only within therapeutic relational spaces (Rosenberg, 1997). My capacity to act is left spinning in an on-going discussion regarding the legitimacy of my need, how need positions me within masculine and feminine dichotomies and the possibility of having my needs met within normative relational boundaries.

3. Above All Make It Look Normal

I sit scrutinizing pictures of my family. In every photograph my parents' bodies pull away from contact with each other, their eyes look in different directions[24]. In group shots with my parents and siblings, I am separate, apart. None of our eyes look the same way. How eloquently our feelings about being together are revealed as we play out looking like a happy family.

Normative relationships contain a sense of fragmentation and entrapment for me, as if there is both no escape and little sustained connection. Remembered qualities, gestures, phrases, bring people towards me in a rush of affection that lasts over time, over memory. Little remains constant in my relationships but my struggle to trust, my sense of aloneness, my longing for connection, and the on-going negotiation of changing lives, priorities, emotions, moods and needs. The legacy I carry, of the public face of my "normal" family and its complete refusal to be accountable to me for its actions, leaves me alone in a confusing quagmire of reality and illusion within relationships, making trust difficult.

I can see myself as a young child standing in the hall with its hard surfaces and slippery floors listening, feeling my insides dissolve, fragment. The scotch tape reassembled each morning to hold me together didn't always stick.

I wake often as an adult, as I did as a child, staring at the ceiling, feeling nothing, wondering how to assemble the energy for another day.

Everyday life becomes a performance, a containment of my inner reality forged in that hallway of my childhood. Mostly I live in a carefully juggled regulation of expectations. I perform the face expected in my family. Fear of misjudgment, humiliation, and hurt, as well as anger, sit somewhere in the background.

This on-going pattern of masking my inner feelings to maintain the face of normativity leaves me hypersensitive to differences between what I perceive and what I am told. The habit of reading the sub-text in relationship (regardless of how inaccurate it may be) makes trust difficult, due to the degree of consistency required[25]. What I face in relationships now is the need to learn conditions in which trust and tolerance of inconsistency become possible. Self-awareness and discipline are required to use the knowledge derived from reading the sub-text of relationship, without reacting protectively in distrust and withdrawal. My need for consistency makes it difficult for me to tolerate ambiguity and leaves me longing to reproduce relations of domination through a fixed, consistent "object" to mirror my "subject".

I sometimes wonder how to tell when my reactions are not only reflective of the performance expected of me within normative frameworks of family, professionalism, motherhood, friendship, and intimate relationships. I want a mantra to hang onto which delineates some possibility beyond normative performance. I know I am not performing my family when my physical boundaries are treated with respect, when I am able to speak about what lies behind the mask, when what I say is not ignored, when my energy goes into myself, not only survival, when I don't hate where I am. It has taken me years to learn this. Most of the time, I still forget and relive the performance. Knowing that others, relating to me in a professional capacity, care for me beyond the dictates of their professional responsibilities helps expand my trust beyond what my performance requires.

As I look at pictures of my children and I, or pictures of us with family friends, our bodies touch, arms link, our eyes share a common direction. I am reassured that there is a difference from the past. If my children have lived beside my sorrow and pain as I have remembered the past, they have not existed in the isolation I experienced. The past is not being entirely repeated. Part of me wonders if this is just a different kind of performance and hopes the clear appearance of affection extends beyond a normative portrait of a happy family.

My husband's establishment in life defined our life together. I was an adored child, responsible as a wife and mother, but not as an adult living my own life. Although we shared decision-making in everyday life and

*talked all the time, there was no communication about the deeper
struggles within our lives. When change came and the limits of our contracts
with one another become visible, there was no room for change.*

*Life-long relationships are sustained through compromise, establishing
habits and expectations and unspoken contracts about how and what
we will be to one another. In the subject-object construction of desire,
what must be forgotten to go on?*

As a child, my relationships with family were designed primarily to meet
my parents' needs. Champagne describes this relationship as "covert incest"
in which the child's desire becomes focused on the needs of the parent
(1996:98,99). Forgetting the feelings of anger and shame that accompany
being used as an object, as well as one's desire as a subject, are fundamental
ways in which this relationship is sustained. Champagne maintains that
"remembering trauma is less about cognitive thinking than about letting go
of defense mechanisms" (1996:110). As a survivor, I am haunted by this
question: what do I continue to deny about the conditions of my life in
order to ensure my survival? My commitment to experience my body and
feelings reduces my capacity to sustain denial once it becomes conscious.
Some of the volatility Herman describes relates to the struggle between the
denial required to sustain relationships, and the dangers of doing so. (1992)

From this perspective, the survivor's task is not one of reentering "normal"
relationships but of constructing possibilities for relationships which move
out of normative subject-object construction. Benjamin (1988) argues for
an incorporation of masculine and feminine characteristics within the self.
Seeing how fundamental the masculine-feminine dichotomy is within
normative discourse, Davies (1990) disagrees with Benjamin. She argues,
instead, for moving away from a masculine-feminine gender dichotomy.
This assumes the characteristics of the other maintain the dichotomy and
do not move towards the potential of multiplicity. Efforts to take on
characteristics from the opposite side of the dichotomy will still be read
and regulated through gendered eyes. Building on the work of Kristeva,
Davies outlines the possibility of a third position, beyond those presented
by liberal or radical feminism:

A move towards an imagined possibility of "woman as whole",
not constituted in terms of the male/female dualism. Such a
move involves confronting one's own personal identity with its

own organization of desire around "masculinity" or "femininity". The desired end point of such a confrontation is to de-massify maleness and femaleness – to reveal their multiple and fragmented nature and remove from the meaning of maleness and femaleness any sense of opposition, hierarchy, or necessary difference. This is not a move towards sameness but towards multiple ways of being. (Davies, 1990: 502)

Game (1991) outlines how desire has been reconceptualized by Cixous as a process of becoming, and by Irigaray as the capacity to be with self and other simultaneously. Along with Davies' fracturing of normative gendered positionings, these conceptions of desire imply a capacity to hold longing or incompletion as part of experience and to engage with the "other" at the same time. Desire without the domination between subject and object becomes a possibility. As an incest survivor seeking to live desire from a subject position, these reconceptions of desire create a possibility for relationship that is not linked to normative patterns of dominance and subjugation.

Towards Living Subject to Subject

The French feminist conception of desire as becoming, as well as Davies' discussion of the dissolving of genders into multiplicity, offer potential to break out of the gendered subject-object dichotomy upon which normative desire rests. Moving towards relationships based on subject-subject positionings within differences in power and privilege seems like a first step out of gendered subject-object relations. Because subject-object relations are dominant, I believe there are only moments of subject to subject relationships. Recognizing how the individual in the object position is also a subject leads to new thinking on this front.

An initial question in the desire to break out of gendered dichotomies relates to how social regulation is lived within the self. If the rational adult is the part of me which maintains normativity, then how do I listen to and understand multiple layers of self?

July 21, 1997
Sitting in therapy last night overwhelmed by the hurt I feel in relationships, how used, how abandoned I feel. All the ways I have been taught to be respectable, to care for others, to understand a different point of view, to meet people half way, to accommodate, leave me feeling like an object. Without becoming a subject, someone others will consider, there is not much point in continuing. It hurts too much.

The question becomes who do I listen to inside, to be a subject in my life? Is it the hurt, outraged three-year-old Sandra Butler believes in? I'm not sure how to take her angry energy and create possibilities that are beyond her concrete capacity to think. Perhaps desires which are not reinforced by normativity live as ambiguous feminine "others", making agency difficult. At the same time, I appear to be developing some experience with subject/subject relations, particularly in relation to my children.

My daughter was born breech, weighing four pounds after an unsettled pregnancy. Although I was allowed to breast feed her, she spent two weeks in an incubator stabilizing her weight and temperature control. When she came home she ate often and cried with colic. At a year she weighed twelve pounds, a perfect replica of her tiny, wiry Welsh ancestry. During her first two years she had frequent ear infections and pneumonia once. As she wasn't the kind of child who went everywhere easily, planning to help her adapt in new situations kept me on edge, as did her health. Until she could talk, I found it hard to judge what her body needed in terms of warmth.

Once she was mobile, she was a tumbling ball of energy emptying cupboards, toy boxes, exploring, learning. I was determined not to break her spirit. My energy went into keeping her safe and building routines to channel her energy. Once she talked much of her energy came out in conversation and then for years in intense relationships with other children. It has only been in recent years that she can tolerate being in the car for any length of time or a dinner time that is later than the norm.

It would have been easy to rage at all the ways (in her differences from me) that I found her difficult and to dictate that she perform according to my priorities and preferences. But it would have been wrong. My life would be diminished without her being all of who she is and all I have learned from her.

My daughter has helped me learn the discipline of love, the creation of structures and boundaries allowing my affection and enjoyment of her energy and enthusiasm for life; allowing us to live openly in our connection. At different times in our life together, this has required different disciplines, to enforce the rules under hot opposition, to keep my opinions strictly to myself, to be honest with her, and to listen and change in accordance with her changes. The richness of our connection has been built and maintained through discipline.

The Role of Discipline in Love

The role of discipline in love is very much about how to use power to create a subject-subject relationship. Authoritarian power demands obedience to the wishes of the more powerful person. Negotiated power assumes a subject-subject relationship and seeks the middle ground. Part of this power is clarifying the purpose of the relationship and creating respect for limits. For example, the parent-child relationship is intended to provide protection and care for the child. The parent's responsibility is to get their primary emotional and physical needs met by peers. While the parent's role is to protect and be present to the child who is a subject, the child must in turn respect what the parent requires as a subject to maintain their protection and care. In describing a reformulated conception of motherhood Benjamin says "the possibility of balancing the recognition of the child's needs with the assertion of one's own has scarcely been put forward as an ideal" (1988: 82). What I have discovered is that the balance between self and other go hand in hand. Benjamin supports this perspective when she describes how children learn of their separateness and gain their autonomy by asserting their will in the presence of another. She says:

> . . . if the other retaliates or caves in and withdraws, we don't really experience the other as outside us . . . A power struggle is inaugurated, and the outcome is a reversible cycle of doer and done to. If the mother does not survive, a pattern is established in which there is no real other subject, no real feeling for the other. (1995: 91)

With self-awareness, thought and patience, the boundary between the child's and parent's needs is negotiated and can respond to change. While this definition of the parent-child relationship is at least given lip service within progressive normative social discourse, the redefinition of the intentions and boundaries of other kinds of relationships based on a subject-subject basis remains an open question for me. Perhaps an on-going way to examine these intentions and boundaries is through the need for accountability, another aspect of the discipline of love.

Seeing my children's displeasure when I was not consistent and accountable for my actions, I decided I needed to change. Becoming more accountable and consistent was more difficult than I imagined. Given the lack of accountability within my own family and the indirectness of their communication, I resisted when I didn't particularly feel like following through. This often happened when I was out having fun and would return an hour later than I said I would without having called. Other times, I would make a promise to do something and then get too busy, or complain about following through or suggest vague plans that would not happen. Realizing my actions had an impact on them helped me learn consistency and accountability. It has also given me the capacity to ask it of them. It has dramatically changed the quality of my relationships.

August 18, 1997

For the first time, I am seeing the contrast between the denial and manipulation that underlie relationships with my family and how I am treated by my friends and my children. For the most part my friends make time for me, communicate the need to make changes in plans, consult me about the changes and do not resort to excusing their behaviour. I am not left through their manipulation to make what feels like impossible choices or feel stabbed in the back. Contact with them does not leave me feeling impotent, angry and hurt. My family takes me to a bleak world where the most minor expectations cannot be counted on. Alive emotionally, my encounters with them teach me about the isolation and emotional chaos where I grew up. What is consistent is my hurt, anger and how, until recently, I have exempted them from "normative" expectations I hold in other relationships.

At the same time, I have reenacted the drama of no accountability and consistency in relationships with others through choosing people who desired more than I could give, and implying more commitment than I could honestly deliver. I can see the gritty discipline of learning to be accountable and consistent in relationships that are important to me. At the current time this struggle is lived in failing to communicate necessary changes in plans. "Forgetting" and procrastinating help me avoid being caught between the needs of my children and the wishes of my partner. The pattern of living silently and very much alone, even in the presence of others, is also present here.

Through this work, the possibility of decent treatment seems greater, and my "read" on the level of inconsistency and betrayal I encounter is more variegated and accurate. The world seems somewhat safer, with more possibilities to establish some trust.

Becoming more accountable and sustaining it requires honesty with yourself and others. This discipline has dramatically shifted the priorities in my life. Words such as duty and obligation have much less pull on my time and energy. My capacity for critical reflection has increased as I live less in states of denial. Although terror and shame accompanied my striving towards honesty rather than toward the normative performance of "niceness", it has helped me count on and trust in the honesty of those close to me.

Sustaining the discipline asked of me by my children has pushed me to become a subject in relation to them and within close friendships. This move towards accountability between subjects contains some capacity to incorporate the inevitability of change. The goal becomes to sustain connection through change "by negotiating conflict and establishing a shared sense of reality – in which one has a sense of agency and impact" (Benjamin, 1995:92).

> *I used to think that love grew through openness. I have longed for a relationship of infinite openness that would surround and incorporate the pain with which I live. The conditions that lead to openness all seem to be about limits and boundaries. Perhaps I am coming to see that no relationship in the world will address the enormous amount of pain with which I live. At best it can be touched or eased in the presence of another. I find this a hard lesson. I would rather not live with this kind of pain, fear and shame. With more acceptance comes more hope, more capacity to reach for the moments of connection and beauty*[26].

In normative relationships, satisfaction of a subject's desire depends on the availability of the object. Increasingly, in my relationship with myself, my children and my friends, I am seeing that my needs are my own. What I actually require or can offer others is much less than I desire. I can offer support through empathy or concrete action, but the depth of another's needs are not mine to address nor are mine their's. This leaves me with more possibilities for being a subject within my own life. My availability is not the sole option others have to get their needs met. With more autonomy, I am freer to give from an open-hearted place of love rather than out of a sense of requirement or obligation. My presence comes from a place of love. By assuming more responsibility for my needs, I am more able to withdraw from the captivity of the subject-object relational dynamic and relate subject to subject. Subject to subject relationships are about moments of affection, feeling connected within the limits defined by each subject. Negotiating relationships based on what is livable for each subject becomes the work.

Sustaining Discipline in Love
The capacity to maintain a subject position ultimately depends on shifting normative relations of power and privilege. The insidious trauma in daily

life of hierarchical subject-object relational constructions undoes the construction of a mutual subject position.(Root in Brown, 1995) Holding onto the subject position in yourself and others is difficult work, particularly in the face of on-going pain. It results in only moments of connectedness, of feeling loved.

From the horrors of the past my children called me towards life seeking connection, recognition and pleasure. They kept me moving through the demands of everyday life, building a home that was different from where I grew up.

> *On good days I embrace this family as a gritty place to live, full of conflict, their changes, my changes, complaints, moments of closeness, shared activities, some laughter. On hard days I wonder how much I do listen, how deep the patterns of denial and silence continue in me, what it means for them to have lived with a parent working through layers of terror and grief. We rarely speak of the incest that formed my life and yet it lives with us. I wonder how much I have resisted commercialism, how much I have encouraged them to think critically. Mostly I feel unseen, taken for granted, rarely "enough", deeply loved and that this is where they are at and need to be.*

> *My choice is to rail at the limits and responsibilities of this relationship, to discount the affection that is here or to accept and let their love in.*

My capacity to sustain myself as both a subject and a parent in the partiality of this relationship depends on my being held elsewhere. I am aware of all the layers which help me maintain the mutuality of subject positions. There is sufficient time, energy, and income to do this work. My white, middle-class privilege supports my image of myself as a subject. There is access to social institutions such as alternative schools which reinforce the combination of freedom and responsibility underpinning the subject position. Although this may once again reflect my feminine gender positioning, I feel most sustained in a daily way by the power of feminist friendship and therapy.

Both feminist therapy and friendship share an understanding of the oppression of women's lives and a commitment to ending those conditions of oppression. Attention is placed on a woman's responsibility to herself rather than on her responsibilities to others. Daring to dream beyond the confines of the normative position becomes possible.

Feminist friendships have given me spaces to be heard into speech, to receive honest feedback and support in risking the actions of becoming a subject. Discipline is required to sustain the capacity for engagement with one another by holding our boundaries, the separateness of our lives, and our capacity to hear one another and respond honestly without judgement. I am surprised at how far I have been carried by the power of listening and support. Although when this power is present it seems magical, it requires hard work to maintain the boundaries which make it possible.

Feminist therapy has provided a much deeper space for the recovery of myself than feminist friendship can hold.

> *My therapist became a rock planted in the middle of my life as I left my marriage, went back to school, struggled at work, with children, in relationships, with house repairs and opened up the terrors, the memories of the past.*

> *I don't know how someone commits to sitting beside someone else's life faithfully at least one hour a week plus telephone calls, to descending into their pit of hell. I'm just glad she did. It has been a long gritty struggle to know and be known.*

For the first time in my life, someone consistently listened and connected to the parts of me which had become masked in order to ensure my survival. There was finally someone who could help me sort through the avalanche of terror, grief, anger and self-hate which lay behind the mask; to slowly come to terms with my actions and responsibilities in the past and in the present. My therapist's willingness to be there, her determination to hear and support what has been lost, affirms my desire to engage with the parts of me behind my mask and to live as a subject. The entrenchment of my self-hate loosens as I let her in genuine affection. This allows new possibilities to grow. But my ability to hold myself in my present life as a subject remains fragile, requiring her support.

Holding Desire
In subject-object relations, desire is conceptualized as providing an impetus towards agency, towards satisfaction. In subject-subject relations, desire is held. Its satisfaction depends on negotiation, not domination. This holding of desire acts as a reflection of the self and the specific conditions of one's life. There is the potential for critical reflection and for less control than in

the formulaic conscription of desire within normative relations. In accepting
the partiality of realizing my desire, I move towards acceptance of what life
brings, without becoming embroiled in the self-hate of the object position.
I long for a normative story that will break the dichotomy, that will affirm
aloneness, separateness, within the power and joy of connection; to replace
the dominant story of completion through love.

In the aloneness of existence, its everyday experiences of violences and
the partiality of human connection, the question of how and where I hold
hope, the aliveness of my life beyond sustaining my endurance, moves to
the forefront. There are only fleeting answers.

*The moments of knowing I am held within a universe are glimpsed
dimly, sometimes joyously and sometimes not at all. They come most
often in nature, the falling leaves, the softening of the light, the silence
of a snowfall, the blossoms each spring. Eliot's still point, the moments
of grace which lift imperfection towards life.*

*I see around me the daily commitments to foster life in the planting of
gardens, the patient care of children, the efforts to create respect and trust
in a violent world.*

*Those who have thought more spiritually for longer say I must learn to
be. Ever my father's daughter I ask what will happen, what will I be able
to do if I learn to be? Will I die well? Learning to be means being in my
body, alive, close to the pain, home.*

Chapter 7

LIVING BESIDE

As I sit here, at the end of a long process that enabled me to articulate the impact of discourses of normativity on my life after the return of incest memories, I wonder about the possibilities for change opened by this work. My work was and is possible because of the hard work of feminists to raise the visibility and credibility of violences against women and children as an issue. However, the nightly newscast continues to record the invisible war against women and children. Another woman dies of assault today as one did yesterday and the day before that. The files I review as part of my job in human services note that approximately one half the girls are survivors of violence. Like me, they may also learn to weave between the fragments left from violation. In the face of the real legacies of my violation and the continued indifference to violence against women and children, what is the work that needs to be done, where is the hope?

On Normativity
Like others with an interest in trauma, I have argued that traumatic experience profoundly shapes the life experience of the individual (Herman, 1992). In therapeutic terms, the on-going imprint of trauma within an individual's life is understood in terms of pathology, as "other" to the "norm". The individual's work is to return to normal. Within this therapeutic framework the survivor's life is reduced to overcoming traumatic experience. All the ways survivors live facets of "normal" life – as friends, mothers, workers and neighbours – may be missed.

By locating the source of the problem solely within the individual, the struggles survivors experience through the impact of "insidious trauma" – patterns of race, class and gender positionings within normative discourses and the underlying violence which helps maintain those patterns – remains invisible. The survivor's everyday life occurs in a social context of on-going violation which compounds the struggle to construct a meaningful existence, and to create on-going relationships and regular patterns of nourishment and sleep.

Normative discourses, which shape individual desires and priorities, also compound the survivor's struggle. Normative discourses of heterosexual monogamy, family, gender and body have all been, and continue to be, sites of both desire and betrayal within my life. Building a life within my ambiguous relationship to these normative discourses increases my sense of "difference" and contributes to my despair.

By articulating how discourses of normativity position my life as an incest survivor, I find the amount of self-blame I generate, when my life does not "return to normal" or when my "symptoms" remain troublesome, is greatly reduced. Understanding discourses of normativity illuminates the idealized portrait of a "normal" life as well as its regulatory power.[27] I have a more solid understanding of how social relations of power and privilege contradict my efforts to live in an embodied way and resist my points of view. The impact of "insidious trauma" on my everyday life is more visible – if frequently overwhelming – and my "deviation" from normative discourses of heterosexual monogamy and family feel more life-giving, with less sense of loss.

Understanding how I am regulated by normative discourses allows me more flexibility, more possibilities to weave differently in and between normative discourses. I can redefine my responsibilities towards family members and the terms of my engagement within relationships, as well as make daily decisions to create a life that will support, rather than shatter, my embodiment. At the same time, my location within social relations will both limit and create these possibilities, and negotiating my way within normative discourses will continue.

Redefining the dominant narrative of incest survivors' experiences from its location in individual pathology towards insidious trauma highlights the social practices through which violence is sustained. The visibility of survivors' daily struggles to live beside the violation, rather than "return to normal", may also make the costs of violence more visible and violence less tolerable. Shattering the normative framework that positions violation in the past and insists recovery is possible creates an opportunity to reconstitute social responsibility to include the present ways in which social relations of domination create violation.

What interests me are the possibilities embodied in refusing the regulatory power of normative discourses, and the spaces that can be created between discourses. Having articulated the impact of normative discourses on my experience as an incest survivor and the construction of my life as "other" to the norm, my sense of shame is reduced. Understanding how normative discourses position their lives as "other" and impact on their everyday experiences, and refusing to be defined in these terms, will help survivors learn to live beside the violation. Therapy which links individual struggles to the social context and which refuses to define incest survivor experiences in terms of pathology and recovery as a return to "normal", can support this work. As the lesson of feminist therapy demonstrates, care and vigilance are required to maintain the critical edge within therapeutic practice.

Survivors and those who support their work need to grapple with the tension between collective social action against violence, and the individualizing and consuming nature of the therapeutic process. Both projects are important and need to happen. Armstrong (1994) eloquently illustrates how the balance has tipped towards the therapeutic. Understanding the power dynamics of this shift is key to developing further social action.

Possibilities also exist to expand the refusal of normative discourses beyond the realm of individual lives. Joan Phillip (1988) describes how the increased visibility of family violence as an issue warranting state intervention creates a dual impact. While greater conformity to normative regulation may result, questions regarding the social viability of the family are also raised. If acceptable narratives of incest survivors' experiences shift to an acknowledgement of "insidious trauma" and the impossibility of ever regaining a "normal" life, the practices which sustain violence may also be highlighted and become less acceptable. Similarly, on-going acknowledgement in the public sphere of living beside violence on a daily basis may also bring greater visibility to the costs of violence and decrease tolerance for it.

In her analysis of discourses of rape, Sharon Marcus (1992) highlights how rape depends on normative frameworks of gender, on domination and violence being played out through the actions, and on the beliefs and conditioning of the individuals involved. In women's refusal to play their part in the normative story, Marcus sees potential to enhance violence prevention, to interrupt the intimidation and to fight back. Claiming a body that can fight, a woman moves towards what Davies describes as breaking gender into "multiple ways of being" (1990: 502). Work which consciously interrupts normative expectations of children, families and women, can contribute to safety and prevention.

Flax describes the challenge to be undertaken when she says:

> To take responsibility is to firmly locate ourselves within contingent and imperfect contexts, to acknowledge differential privileges of race, gender, geographical location, and sexual

identities, and to resist the delusionary and dangerous hope of redemption in a world not of our own making. We need to learn to make claims on our own and others' behalf and to listen to those which differ from ours, knowing that ultimately there is nothing that justifies them beyond each person's own desire, and need and the discursive practices in which these are developed, embedded, and legitimated. Each person's well-being is ultimately dependent on the development of discursive communities which foster (among other attributes) an appreciation of and desire for difference, empathy, even indifference in the others. Lacking such feelings, as the Jews in Germany or people of color in the United States (among many others) have discovered, all the laws and culture civilization can offer will not save us. (1992: 460)

The strategy used throughout this work, of articulating places of discomfort and silence – which may first register in the body – as a building block in understanding how relations of power and privilege are constructed in everyday life, may begin to move towards Flax's vision.

Within the complexity of what must be undertaken, the needs are clear. Social responses towards childhood sexual abuse, neglect and poverty are a travesty of what children need and deserve. Discourses which foreground the importance of family and permit children to grow up in poverty and live in conditions of abuse and neglect require challenging not only in the legislature but in our actions, beliefs and practices. The discourses in and through which our lives are constructed have an impact – if differently – on us all. Who is listening and to what?

Long term solutions require dismantling normative systems of power and privilege based on power over. Individual courage and institutional supports to shift normative expectations of gender and family contribute to these efforts. Working in and between discourses, like Valverde's "green shopper", offers possible first steps. Education which links childhood sexual abuse to normative frameworks of power and privilege, rather than replicating the therapeutic perspective of dysfunction, may contribute to diminishing denial, thereby increasing social commitment to child protection. Similarly, linking perpetrators' understanding of their actions to the normative gendering of boys and men may also further educational efforts. Issues feminists have fought for in order to create possibilities for autonomy and independence for women – pay equity, child care, reproductive control, protection from harassment and violence – remain key for the protection of children.

The capacity to live in and between discourses depends on recognizing fluidity, rather than immobility, within discourses. How experience is understood is constantly being regulated and resisted. The task is to take up the challenge of critical engagement with desires, beliefs and practices in normative discourses, and not replicate dominant expectations.

Living Beside

The questions I am asking now are different from those I asked when I began this project. This does not signal my healing or my return to "normal". Learning to live beside the violation currently occupies my attention similar to the ways weaving between the fragments did throughout the development of this work.

The possibilities for living alive lie somewhere between the constructions of the dichotomies of public and private, risk and safety, alive and numb. Living beside the violation means finding ways to acknowledge the on-goingness of it; to risk safely in ways that will not catapult me into past captivity. It also means accepting the limits of what is tolerable, knowing how risk brings terror. The normative standards of success which my father reproduced for me may not, in fact, be the only possibility or the most satisfying option.

Living beside the violation, finding hope is troublesome. Do I dare to hope once again? According to *The Winston Dictionary*, hope is characterized by elements of desire and trust. What I encountered early in life was desire and betrayal. What and how to trust are key questions in terms of finding possibilities for hope.

The capacity for trust requires an acceptance of fluidity, change and partiality. In many ways, what I have hoped for in the past is the static flip-side of captive relations. It is a place where I will at last be safe, where the struggle will be over, where I will know what I want and will be able to achieve it, where my life will be balanced and love and attention will be readily available. What I experience in myself and others is not the consistency of my desires, attention or affection, but its partiality and fluidity, making trust in myself and others difficult.

My therapist repeatedly tells me to trust the process. While I sense she is right, the shape and form of what is to be trusted eludes me. Perhaps it is trust in my own survival, in my abilities to risk and retreat as required. Part of what must be risked is a tolerance for ambiguity, in which normative patterns are broken, and the end of the story is no longer predictable. My ability to risk is hampered by fear of being hurt and betrayed, fear of being stupid. It is clearer to me that regardless of what I do someone is bound to think it's pretty stupid. Oddly enough, this leaves me with a sense of freedom; it pushes beyond the social expectations embodied in my father to get it right. That I will be hurt and betrayed is a certainty. Perhaps it is knowing and trusting I will survive the hurt and betrayal that makes risk possible. Nonetheless, the formative legacy of hurt leaves me self-protective and struggling to maintain a separation between present and past. Maintaining trust in myself and others requires on-going support to hold my ground, to separate from the conditions of the past. I see how quickly erosion in my abilities to trust myself and others begins; tiny doubts become a slippery slope back into the silence and obedience of captivity.

Learning to live beside the violation is now the centre of my struggle. I continue to understand that the trauma of the past remains an immutable part of what forms me. I slip easily back into the terror and survival patterns of the past. But this is not all of who I am. If I shattered, standing in the hallway of my childhood, and I carry that shattered self with me today, I also walked out of that hallway and became who I am today, which is more than that shattering[28]. With the reception of this work in the public realm, the contradictions between how I learned to understand myself in the past and how I am now are obvious, even to me. The struggle has become one of holding a different sense of self than the one learned early on. This, in turn, requires clearly accepting that the patterns of relationships in my family were crazy.

Living beside means acknowledging the traumatized parts of self as they arise in daily life. It means honouring them and giving them space for expression. As soon as I resist and refuse these parts of myself, I quickly move back into relationships and a sense of self that reflect past patterns of survival. When I honour the trauma, I gain the flexibility to move into different parts of myself to create new possibilities. I work to strengthen my capacity to hear and affirm messages in the present which speak of competence, affection and hope. What I have learned, through traumatic experience, is to listen to messages of impending danger and inadequacy. It is sometimes possible to hear, dream and act as if life beyond survival is a possibility. But I am aware of the long road it took to get here, the ton of courage, understanding and affection it has taken to create the possibility of standing on a different relational platform within myself and with others, and the continued fragility with which hope is held.

A child called Henrietta has danced through my imagination during the past year. I wonder why this child has appeared now; what it is I need to hear and to listen for? She is the child I long to have been, not the child I was. To the extent that I can imagine her and bring her to life, her spirit and energy are alive in me. Henrietta dislikes formal structure, routine and under-handed power plays. She is energetic, curious, off to explore the world, determined to live in it, to be a part of it rather than watch it. She is disruptive, irreverent or absent in the face of boredom or pomposity. Henrietta's energy, clarity and determination awake my own and her sense that anything is possible lives inside me momentarily.

Having reached middle age, the people around me who will die young are now beginning to do so. The ordinary activities of life which I take for granted at times carry an element of privilege and gratitude. To the extent that it will ever be possible, the time to break patterns of the past, to incorporate the knowledge of trauma differently into my life and to embrace the gift of Henrietta, is now.

NOTES

1. My thanks to Sharon Rosenberg for her insight into the importance of discourses of normativity as the central framework for this text.
2. For an interesting discussion on a child's desire for sex with an adult see Alcoff (1996) "The Politics of Pedophilia" in *Feminist Interpretations of Foucault*. S. Hekman (ed.) Penn.: State University Press. She concludes "I believe that the dangers of adult-child sex are significant enough to warrant a general prohibition" (129).
3. Suggested changes in legislation currently being considered by the Ontario government would create additional grounds to strengthen child protection.
4. The phrase insidious trauma is derived from Root (1992).
5. Elizabeth Kelly (1987) refers to a continuum of violence. However, I think that the parallel can be made to experiences of captivity. My thanks to Marilyn Vivian for helping me to clarify this point.
6. My questions of what I am responsible for and to whom echo this historical emphasis on the patient's taking responsibility for his/her actions.
7. For an interesting discussion on the use of statistics to establish "facts" about women in the mental health system see D. Smith (1990). While she supports an analysis of the gendered power imbalances within the mental health system, Smith demonstrates that statistical information changes depending on what is included and excluded.
8. See also Jennings (1994) for an excellent discussion of the effects of psychotropic medication and the revictimizing impact of psychiatric care for her daughter who was a survivor of childhood sexual abuse.
9. For a more comprehensive discussion of survivor writing see Janice Williamson "Writing Aversion" in *By, For and About: Feminist Cultural Politics*. Wendy Waring (ed) Toronto: Women's Press, 1994.
10. I want to acknowledge survivor accounts which do not fall into this therapeutic framework. These include Danica (1988; 1996), Warland (1990) and Bulkin (1990). Danica's recent work, like that of Bulkin and Warland, describes survivor experiences within the context of everyday life rather than emphasizing the therapeutic process.
11. This work has now been published as *The Trouble with Normal: Postwar Youth and the Making of Heterosexuality*. Toronto: University of Toronto Press, 1997.
12. My thanks to Marilyn Vivian for pointing this out.

13. Feminist theorists would outline my mother's economic vulnerability, and the social "legitimation" of my father's dominance (Elliot, 1996)
14. My thanks to Kari Dehli for pointing this out to me.
15. My thanks to Kari Dehli for this example.
16. My thanks to Kari Dehli for adding this layer.
17. My thanks to Kari Dehli for clarifying this point.
18. My thanks to Kari Dehli for articulating this insight.
19. Kari Dehli, personal communication, 1997.
20. Kari Dehli, personal communication, 1997.
21. My thanks to Kari Dehli for making this link to Judith Butler.
22. Kari Dehli, personal communication, 1997.
23. My thanks to Kari Dehli for pointing this out.
24. This technique of examining photographs came from a workshop held in Oct., 1996 in Toronto by Rosie Martin. My thanks to her.
25. At the same time valuable information is obtained through reading the sub-text (see Chapter 2)
26. This focus on relationship as a vehicle to alleviate pain reflects my feminine gender positioning. Other endeavours such as creativity contain possibilities for remaking individual experience. This in turn moves towards breaking open the gender dichotomy towards multiplicity (Davies, 1990). My thanks to Ann Decter for pointing this out.
27. My thanks to Kari Dehli for pointing this out.
28. My thanks to Marilyn Struthers for helping me see this.

Bibliography

Abbott, F. (1993) "Introduction Reclaiming Boyhood and Saving Our Lives" in F.Abbott (ed.) *Boyhood: Growing Up Male A Multicultural Anthology*. Freedom CA.: Crossing Press.

Acker, S. & Feuerverger, G. (1996) "Doing Good and Feeling Bad, The Work of Women University Teachers" in *Cambridge Journal of Education*, Vol. 26, #3.

Adams, Mary Louise (1994) "The Trouble with Normal: Postwar Youth and the Construction of Heterosexuality" Unpublished PhD Thesis, University of Toronto.

Alcoff, Linda (1996) "Dangerous Pleasure: Foucault and the Politics of Pedophilia" in S.Hekman (ed.) *Feminist Interpretations of Michel Foucault* Pennsylvania: Pennsylvania State University.

Alcoff, Linda & Gray, Laura (1993) "Survivor Discourse: Transgression or Recuperation?" in *Signs: Journal of Women in Culture and Society.* Vol. 18, No. 21.

Antze, Paul & Lambek, Michael (1996) *Tense Past: Cultural Essays in Trauma and Memory*. New York: Routledge.

Armstrong, Louise (1994) *Rocking the Cradle of Sexual Politics: What Happened When Women Said Incest*. Reading, Mass.: Addison Wesley.

Armstrong, Louise (1983) *The Home Front: Notes from the Family War Zone*. New York: McGraw-Hill.

Backus, John & Stannard, Barbara (1994) "Your Memories Are Not False A Reply to the False Memory Foundation". Distributed by Survivorship, San Francisco, CA.

Bass, Ellen & Davis, Laura. (1988) *The Courage to Heal: A Guide for Women Survivors of Child Sexual Abuse*. New York: Harper & Row.

Bellamy, Elizabeth J. & Leontis, Artemis. (1993) "A Genealogy of Experience: From Epistemology to Politics" in *The Yale Journal of Criticism*, Vol. 6, No. 1, p.163-184.

Benjamin, Jessica (1995) *Like Subjects, Like Objects: Essays on Recognition and Sexual Difference.* New Haven: Yale University.

Benjamin, Jessica. (1988) *The Bonds of Love.* New York: Pantheon Books.

Berland, Jody (1993) "Condemned to Meaning: Sex, Gender, Knowledge, Pain" in *Let's Play Doctor: Undoing The Ruse of Clinical Objectivity and its Pathological Placement of the Feminine.* Artspeak Gallery, April 23-May 23, Vancouver, B.C.

Binhammer, K.; Cotnoir, L.; Godard, B.; Henderson, J.; Moyes, Lianne. (1993) "For The Record..." in Tessera. Vol. 14, Summer.

Bishop, Anne (1994) *Becoming An Ally.* Halifax: Fernwood Publishing.

Bordo, Susan R. (1989) "The Body and the Reproduction of Femininity: A Feminist Appropriation of Foucault" in A. Jaggar & S. Bordo (eds.) *Gender Body Knowledge.* New Jersey: Rutgers University Press.

Britzman, Deborah P. (1998) *Lost Subjects, Contested Objects.* Albany, NY: SUNY Press.

Brown, Laura (1995) "Not Outside the Range: One Feminist Perspective on Psychic Trauma" in C. Caruth (ed.) *Trauma: Explorations In Memory.* Baltimore: John Hopkins University Press.

Bulkin, E. (1990) *Enter Password: Recovery.* Albany N.Y.: Turtle Books.

Burstow, Bonnie. (1992) *Radical Feminist Therapy: Working in the Context of Violence,* Newbury Park, CA: Sage Publications.

Burstow, B. & Weitz, D. (1988) *Shrink Resistant: The Struggle Against Psychiatry in Canada.* Vancouver: New Star Books.

Butler, Judith (1990) *Gender Trouble: Feminism and the Subversion of Identity.* New York: Routledge.

Butler, Sandra (1994) "Breaking & Entering: Shattered Trust" Taped workshop presentation from the "It's Never OK" Conference. Toronto: Oct. 13, 1994.

Butler, Sandra (1992) Notes From Public Lecture, OISE & Workshops, Centre for Christian Studies, Toronto, March 23-26.

Butler, Sandra. (1985) *The Conspiracy of Silence.* Volcano, CA.: Volcano Press.

Caplan, Paula (1995) *They Say You're Crazy*. Reading Mass.: Addison-Wesley.

Capponi, Pat (1992) *Upstairs in the Crazy House The Life of a Psychiatric Survivor*. Toronto: Viking Press.

Caruth, Cathy (1995) "Introduction" in Cathy Caruth (ed.) *Trauma Explorations in Memory*. Baltimore, MD: John Hopkins University Press.

Champagne, Rosaria (1996) *The Politics of Survivorship*. New York: New York University Press.

Chang, Elaine K. (1994) "A Not-So-New Spelling of My Name Notes Toward (and Against) a Politics of Equivocation" in Angelica Bammer (ed.) *Displacements: Cultural Identities in Question*. Indianapolis: Indiana University Press.

Chandler, Clarissa, (1990) "Flashbacks, Retrieval, Care & Management". Taped workshop presentation at the "No More Secrets" Conference.

Chandler, Clarissa, (1990) "Identifying Your Own Healing Path" in Regan McClure (ed.) *Loving In Fear*. Toronto: Queer Press.

Chesler, Phyllis, (1972) *Women & Madness*. New York: Doubleday.

Chrystos, (1991) "I'm Burning Up" in *Dream On*. Press Gang.

Church, K.L.(1995) *Forbidden Narratives: Critical Autobiography As Social Science*. U.S.A.: Gordon & Breach.

Corrigan, Philip (1990) *Social Forms/Human Capacities: Essays in Authority and Difference*. London: Routledge.

Culbertson, Roberta (1995) "Embodied Memory, Transcendence, and Telling: Recounting Trauma, Re-establishing the Self" in *New Literary History*, 26:IV, p. 169-195.

Dallery, Arlene B. (1989) "The Politics of Writing (the) Body: Ecriture Feminine" in A. Jaggar & S. Bordo (eds.) *Gender Body Knowledge*. New Jersey: Rutgers University Press.

Danica, Elly, (1996) *Beyond Don't: Dreaming Past The Dark*. Charlottetown, P.E.I.: Gynergy.

Danica, Elly, (1988) *Don't: A Woman's Word*. Charlottetown, P.E.I.: Gynergy.

Davies, Bronwyn (1990) "The Problem of Desire" in *Social Problems*, Vol. 37, #4, Nov.

Davies, Bronwyn (1989) *Frogs and Snails and Feminist Tales.* North Sydney, Australia: Allen & Unwin.

Dehli, Kari (1994) "They Rule by Sympathy: The Feminization of Pedagogy" in M. Valverde (ed.) *Studies in Moral Regulation.* Toronto: Centre of Criminology, University of Toronto.

Donzelot, Jacques (1980) *The Policing of Families.* London: Hutchinson.

Elliot, Faith (1996) "Violence and Sexual Abuse in Family Life" in *Gender, Family and Society.* London: MacMillan Press.

Ellsworth, Elizabeth (1993) "Claiming the Tenured Body" in Delese Wear (ed). *The Center of the Web: Women and Solitude.* State University of New York Press.

Epstein, D. & Johnson, R.(1997) *Schooling Sexualities.* Buckingham: Open University Press.

Ernst, Sheila & Goodison, Lucy. (1985) *In Our Own Hands: A Book of Self-Help Therapy.* London: The Women's Press.

Feldman-Summers, Shirley & Pope, Kenneth S. (1994) "The Experience of "Forgetting Childhood Abuse: A National Survey of Psychologists" in *The Journal of Consulting & Clinical Psychology*, Volume 62, #3, p. 636-639.

Fenwick, P. & Fenwick, E. (1995) *The Truth in the Light: An Investigation of Over 300 Near-Death Experiences.* London: Headline.

Finkler, Lilith (1993) "Notes for Feminist Theorists on the Lives of Psychiatrized Women" in *Canadian Women Studies*, Vol. 13, No. 4, p. 72-74.

Flax, Jane (1993) "Multiples: On the Contemporary Politics of Subjectivity" in *Human Studies*, 16: 33-49.

Flax, Jane (1992) "The End of Innocence" in J. Butler & J. Scott (ed.) *Feminists Theorize the Political.* New York: Routledge.

Flax, Jane (1990) *Thinking Fragments Psychoanalysis, Feminism & Postmodernism in the Contemporary West.* Berkeley, CA: University of California Press.

Flax, Jane (1987) "Re-Membering The Selves: Is The Repressed Gendered?" in *Michigan Quarterly Review,* Vol.XXVI, No.1. Issue on Women and Memory.

Flax, Jane (1986) "Gender As A Problem: In and For Feminist Theory" in *Amerikan Studies/American Studies.*

Forward, S. & Buck, C. (1988) *Betrayal of Innocence.* Harrisonburg,VA: Penguin.

Fraser, Sylvia, (1987) *My Father's House: A Memoir of Incest and of Healing.* Toronto: Doubleday.

Frankenberg, Ruth (1993) *White Women, Race Matters The Social Construction of Whiteness.* Minneapolis: University of Minnesota Press.

Freyd, Jennifer (1996) *Betrayal Trauma.* Cambridge, Mass.: Harvard University Press.

Gahlinger, Claudia (1993) *Woman In The Rock.* Charlottetown, P.E.I.: Gynergy.

Game, Ann (1991) *Undoing the Social Towards a Deconstructive Sociology.* Toronto: University of Toronto Press.

Gerrard, Nikki & Javed, Nayyar (1995) "The Psychology of Women" in *Feminist Issues: Race, Class & Sexuality,* Scarborough: Prentice Hall.

Gilleland, B.E. & James, R.K. (1993) "Posttraumatic Stress Disorder" in *Crisis Intervention Strategies,* Pacific Grove CA.: Brooks/Cole Publishing.

Gilligan, Carol (1982) *In A Different Voice.* Mass.: Harvard University Press.

Goffman, Erving (1963) *Stigma.* Englewood Cliffs N.J.: Prentice Hall.

Gordon, Colin (1980) *Power/Knowledge Selected Interviews and Other Writings* 1972-1977 Michel Foucault. New York:Pantheon.

Greenspan, Miriam (1993) *A New Approach To Women and Therapy.* Blue Ridge Summit PA: McGraw-Hill Second Edition.

Griffiths, Morwenna (1995) *Feminisms and the Self: The Web of Identity.* London: Routledge.

Grosz, Elizabeth (1995) *Space, Time and Perversion: Essays on the Politics of Bodies.* New York: Routledge.

Gunn, Rita & Linden, Rick (1994) "The Processing of Child Sexual Abuse Cases" in *Confronting Sexual Assault: A Decade of Legal and Social Change.* Toronto: University of Toronto Press.

Hacking, Ian (1996) "Memory Sciences, Memory Politics" in P. Antze & M. Lambek (ed.) *Tense Past: Cultural Essays in Trauma and Memory.* New York: Routledge.

Harvey, Mary & Herman, Judith Lewis (1994) "Amnesia, Partial Amnesia & Delayed Recall among Adult Survivors of Childhood Trauma" in *Consciousnesss & Cognition,* Vol.3, p. 295-306.

Haug, Frigga (ed.) (1987) *Female Sexualization.* London: Verso Press.

Health & Welfare Canada (1991) *Family Violence Situation Paper and Backgrounders,* Family Violence Prevention Division.

Health & Welfare Canada (1991) Reaching for Solutions, Report of the Special Advisor on Child Sexual Abuse, National Clearinghouse on Family Violence.

Henriques, J.; Hollway, W.; Urwin, C.; Venn, C.; Walkerdine, V. (1984) *Changing the Subject.* New York: Methuen & Co.

Herman, Judith Lewis (1996) "Crime & Memory" in Charles Strozier & Michael Flynn (eds) *Trauma & Self.* Maryland: Rowan & Littlefield Publishers.

Herman, Judith with Lisa Hirschman (1993) "Father-Daughter Incest" in P.B. Bart & E.G. Moran (ed.) *Violence Against Women: The Bloody Footprints.* Newbury Park CA: Sage.

Herman, Judith Lewis (1992). *Trauma and Recovery.* New York: Basic Books.

Hoppen, Jane (1994) "Trying to Return" in *Feminist Studies,* 20, No. 2, Summer.

Hutchinson, T. (ed) (1961) *Poetical Works of Wordsworth.* London: Oxford University Press.

Jackson, David. (1990) *Unmasking Masculinity: A Critical Autobiography* London: Unwin Hyman

Jacobs, J.L. (1994) *Victimized Daughters: Incest and the Development of the Female Self.* New York: Routledge.

Jacobs, Janet Liebman (1993) "Victimized Daughters: Sexual Violence and the Empathic Female Self" in *Signs,* Vol.19, No.1, p.126-145.

Jaggar, Alison (1989) "Love and Knowledge: Emotion in Feminist Epistemology" in A. Jaggar & S. Bordo (eds.) *Gender Body and Knowledge*. London: Rutgers.

Jennings, Ann & Ralph, Ruth (1997) "In Their Own Words", Maine Trauma Advisory Groups Report. Dept. of Mental Health, Mental Retardation & Substance Abuse Services, Office of Trauma Services.

Jennings, Ann (1994) "On Being Invisible in the Mental Health System" in *The Journal of Mental Health Administration*, Commentary, Vol. 21, No. 4, Fall, p.374-387.

Jordan, Judith (ed.) (1997) *Women's Growth In Diversity*. New York: Guilford Press.

Kadi, Joanna (1996) *Thinking Class Sketches From a Cultural Worker*. Boston, MA: South End Press.

Kaschak, Ellyn (1992) *Engendered Lives A New Psychology of Women's Experience*. New York: Basic Books.

Kaufman, Michael. (1993) *Cracking the Armor Power & Pain in the Lives of Men*. Toronto: Penguin Books.

Kelly, E. (1987) "The Continuum of Sexual Violence" in J. Hanmer & M. Maynard (ed.) *Women Violence and Social Control*. Atlantic Highlands N.J.: Humanities Press.

King, Cathy (1997) "Boys & Us" in *Lesbian Parenting: Living With Pride & Prejudice*. Charlottetown, P.E.I.: Gynergy.

Kinsman, Gary (1987) *The Regulation of Desire, Sexuality in Canada*. Montreal: Black Rose Books.

Kirmayer, Lawrence (1996) "Landscapes of Memory: Trauma, Narrative, and Dissociations" in P. Antze & M. Lambek (ed.) *Tense Past: Cultural Essays in Trauma and Memory*. New York: Routledge.

Kirzner, Ellie (1992) "Power Play" in Now Magazine, Dec, 24-30, p. 12, 13 &19.

Kirzner-Roberts, J. (1992) "Slap Shots Against Boys' Masculinity" in *Now Magazine*, Dec. 24-30, p.13&21.

Kuhn, Annette (1995) *Family Secrets: Acts of Memory and Imagination*. London: Verso Press.

Lasch, Christopher (1977) *Haven in a Heartless World: The Family Besieged.* New York: Basic Books.

Laub, Dori (1995) "Truth and Testimony: The Process and the Struggle" in Cathy Caruth (ed.) *Trauma: Explorations In Memory.* Baltimore, MD: John Hopkins University Press.

Lauretis de, Teresa (1990) "Upping the Anti (sic) in Feminist Theory" in M. Hirsch & E. Fox Keller (eds.) *Conflicts in Feminism.* New York: Routledge.

Lew, M. (1988) *Victims No Longer.* New York: Harper & Row.

Little, Margaret (1994) "Manhunts and Bingo Blabs: The Moral Regulation of Ontario Single Mothers" in M. Valverde (ed.) *Studies in Moral Regulation.* Toronto: Centre of Criminology, University of Toronto.

Lorde, Audre (1984) *Sister Outsider.* Freedom CA: The Crossing Press.

MacDonald, Ann-Marie (1996) *Fall On Your Knees.* Toronto: Alfred A. Knopf.

Marcus, Sharon (1992) "Fighting Bodies, Fighting Words: A Theory and Politics of Rape Prevention" in J. Butler & J. Scott (eds.) *Feminists Theorize the Political* New York: Routledge.

Meiselman, Karen C. (1978) *Incest.* San Francisco: Jossey-Bess Publishers.

Messner, Michael (1992) *Power at Play.* Boston: Beacon Press.

Michaels, Anne (1996) *Fugitive Pieces.* Toronto: McClelland & Stewart.

Miller, Alice (1990) *Banished Knowledge Facing Childhood Injuries.* New York: Doubleday.

Miller, Alice (1981) *The Drama of the Gifted Child.* New York: Harper Collins.

Miller, Jean Baker (1976) *Towards A New Psychology of Women.* Boston: Beacon Press.

Miller, Nancy (1991) *Getting Personal Feminist Occasions & Other Autobiographical Acts.* New York: Routledge.

Millett, K. (1990) *The Loony Bin Trap.* New York: Touchstone.

Mohanty, Chandra Talpade (1987) "Feminist Encounters Locating the Politics of Experience" in *Copyright* 1 Fall, p. 30-44.

Moore, Henrietta (1994) "The Problem of Explaining Violence in the Social Sciences" in P. Harvey & P. Gow (ed.) *Sex and Violence: Issues in Representation*. London: Routledge.

Murray, G. (1993) "Picking on the Little Guy: In Boyhood and on the Battlefield" in F. Abbott (ed.) *Boyhood Growing Up Male A Multicultural Anthology*. Freedom CA.: Crossing Press.

Narayan, Uma (1989) "The Project of Feminist Epistemology: Perspectives from a Nonwestern Feminist" in A. Jaggar & S.Bordo (ed.) *Gender Body & Knowledge*. London: Rutgers.

Narayan, Uma, (1988) "Working Together Across Difference: Some Considerations On Emotions & Political Practice" in *Hypatia,* Vol. 3, No. 2, Summer.

Nathan, Debbie & Haaken, Jan (1996) "From Incest to Ivan the Terrible Science and the Trials of Memory" in *Tikkun,* Sept./Oct.

Orange, Donna (1995) *Emotional Understanding: Studies in Psychoanalytic Epistemology*. New York: Guilford Press.

Parker, Ian; Georgaca, Eugenie; Harper, David; McLaughlin, Terence & Stowell-Smith, Mark. (1995) *Deconstructing Psychopathology*. London: Sage Publications.

Pharr, Suzanne (1988) *Homophobia Weapon of Sexism*. Inverness, CA: Chardon Press.

Phelan, Shane, (1993) "(Be)Coming Out: Lesbian Identity and Politics" in *Signs,* Vol.18, No. 4, p. 765–790.

Phillip, Joan (1988) *Policing The Family: Social Control in Thatcher's Britain*. London: Junius Publications.

Potter, Nancy (1995) "The Severed Head and Existential Dread: The Classroom as Epistemic Community and Student Survivors of Incest" in *Hypatia,* Vol. 10, No. 2, Spring.

Pratt, Minnie Bruce (1991) *Rebellion Essays 1980-1991*. Ithaca: Firebrand Books.

Pratt, Minnie Bruce (1984) "Identity: Skin Blood Heart" in *Yours In Struggle: Three Feminist Perspectives on Anti-Semitism and Racism*. Ithaca: Firebrand Books.

Rabinow, Paul (ed). (1984) *The Foucault Reader.* New York: Pantheon Books.

Randall, Margaret (1987) *This Is About Incest.* Ithaca: Firebrand Books.

Ras, Marion de & Grace, Victoria (eds.) (1997) *Bodily Boundaries, Sexualised Genders and Medical Discourses.* Palmerston North, New Zealand: Dunmore Press.

Renvoize, Jean. (1993) *Innocence Destroyed A Study of Child Sexual Abuse.* London: Routledge.

Rich, Adrienne (1986) "Compulsory Heterosexuality and Lesbian Existence" in *Blood, Bread & Poetry.* New York & London: W. W. Norton.

Rich, Adrienne (1986) "Resisting Amnesia: History and Personal Life" in *Blood, Bread and Poetry.* New York & London: W. W. Norton.

Roberts, J.V. & Mohr, R.M. (1994) *Confronting Sexual Assault A Decade of Legal and Social Change.* Toronto: University of Toronto Press.

Rockhill, Kathleen (1996) "And Still I Fight" in *Canadian Women's Studies,* Vol.16, Number 2, Spring.

Rockhill, Kathleen (1993) "Homecries" in *Tessera,* Vol.14, Summer.

Root, Maria P.P. (1992) "Reconstructing the Impact of Trauma on Personality" in L.S.Brown & M. Ballou (eds.) *Personality and Psychopathology Feminist Reappraisals.* New York: Guilford Press.

Rosenberg, Sharon (1997) "Rupturing the 'Skin of Memory': Bearing Witness to the 1989 Massacre of Women in Montreal". Unpublished PhD Thesis, University of Toronto.

Russell, Diane E.H. (1986) *The Secret Trauma: Incest in the Lives of Girls and Women.* New York: Basic Books.

Schwartz, H. (1993) "Reflections on a Cold War Boyhood" in F. Abbott (ed.) *Boyhood: Growing Up Male A Multicultural Anthology.* Freedom, CA.: Crossing Press.

Scott, Joan W. (1992) "Experience" in J. Butler & J.Scott (eds.) *Feminists Theorize the Political.* London: Routledge.

Seidman, P. (1993) "A Personal Exploration into the Politics of Boyhood" in F. Abbott.(ed.) *Boyhood: Growing Up Male A Multicultural Anthology.* Freedom CA.: Crossing Press.

Sink, Frances (1988) "Sexual Abuse in the Lives of Children" in Martha Straus (ed.) *Abuse and Victimization Across the Life Span*. Baltimore: The John Hopkins University Press.

Silverstein, Olga & Rashbaum, Beth (1994) *The Courage To Raise Good Men*. New York: Viking.

Smith, Dorothy (1990) *The Conceptual Practices of Power: A Feminist Sociology of Knowledge*. Toronto: University of Toronto Press.

Smith, Dorothy (1987) *The Everyday World as Problematic: A Feminist Sociology*. Toronto: University of Toronto Press.

Smith, Dorothy (1975) "Women & Psychiatry" in D. Smith & S. David (eds.) *Women Look At Psychiatry*. Vancouver: Press Gang.

Smith, Margaret (1993) *Ritual Abuse: What is It Why It Happens How To Help*. San Francisco: Harper.

Spence, Jo (1995) *Cultural Sniping: The Art of Transgression*. London: Routledge Press.

Steed, Judy (1994) *Our Little Secret: Confronting Child Sexual Abuse in Canada*. Toronto: Random House.

Steele, Kathy (1987) "Sitting with the Shattered Soul" in *Pilgrimage: Journal of Personal Exploration & Psychotherapy*, Vol. 15 No. 6.

Stern, D.N. (1985) *The Interpersonal World of the Infant*. New York: Basic Books.

Stiver, Irene (1990) "Dysfunctional Families and Wounded Relationships - Part I". Paper presented at a Stone Centre Colloquium, May 3, 1989.

Stiver, Irene. (1990) "Dysfunctional Families and Wounded Relationships - Part II." Paper presented at a Stone Centre Colloquium on November 1, 1989.

Straus, Martha B. (1988) *Abuse and Victimization Across the Life Span*. Baltimore: John Hopkins University Press.

Sullivan, E. (1984) *A Critical Psychology*. New York: Plenum Press.

Sykes, Darlene & Symons-Moulton, Brenda (1991) "Child Abuse" in Suzanne Mulligan (ed.) *A Handbook for the Prevention of Family Violence.* The Family Violence Prevention Project of The Community Child Abuse Council of Hamilton-Wentworth.

Tal, Kali (1996) *Worlds of Hurt.* Cambridge: Cambridge University Press.

Terr, Lenore (1994) *Unchained Memories: True Stories of Traumatic Memories Lost and Found.* New York: Basic Books.

Tompkins, Jane (1989) "Me and My Shadow" in Linda Kaufman (ed.) *Gender and Theory: Dialogues on Feminist Criticism.* Oxford & New York: Blackwell.

Tompkins, Jane (1996) "Let's Get Lost" in H. Arem Veeser (ed.) *Confessions of the Critics.* New York: Routledge.

Valverde, Marianna (ed.) (1994) *Studies In Moral Regulation.* Toronto.: Centre of Criminology, University of Toronto.

Valverde, Marianna (1991) " As If Subjects Existed: Analyzing Social Discourses" in *Canadian Review of Sociology and Anthropology,* Vol.28, #2, May, p.173 - 187.

Van der Kolk, Bessel, A. & Van der Hart, Onno, (1995) "The Intrusive Past: The Flexibility of Memory & The Engraving of Trauma" in C. Caruth, (ed) *Trauma: Explorations In Memory.* Baltimore: John Hopkins University Press.

Van der Kolk, Bessel, A. (1994) "The Body Keeps Score: Memory and the Evolving Psychobiology of Posttraumatic Stress" The Massachusetts General Hospital Trauma Clinic, Harvard Medical School, Boston, Mass.

Venn, Couze (1984) "The Subject of Psychology" in J. Henriques, W. Hollway, C. Urwin, C, Venn, V. Walkerdine *Changing The Subject.* New York: Methuen & Co.

Wakefield, Hollinda & Underwager, Ralph "Magic, Mischief and Memories: Remembering Repressed Abuse". Northfield, MN: Institute for Psychological Therapies.

Walker, Alice (1982) *The Color Purple.* New York: Harcourt, Brace, Jovanovich.

Walkerdine, Valerie (1990) *Schoolgirl Fictions.* New York: Verso.

Walkerdine, Valerie & Lucey, Helen (1989) *Democracy In The Kitchen: Regulating Mothers and Socializing Daughters.* London: Cox & Wyman.

Walkerdine, Valerie (1984) "Developmental Psychology and the Child-Centered Pedagogy: the Insertion of Piaget into Early Education" in J. Henriques; W. Hollway; C. Urwin; C. Venn; V. Walkerdine (eds.) *Changing the Subject.* New York: Methuen.

Wallen, Ruth (1994) "Memory Politics The Implications of Healing From Sexual Abuse in *Tikkun.* Nov./Dec. Vol. 1 9 (6).

Walsh, R. (1990) *The Spirit of Shamanism.* New York: J.P. Tarcher/Putnam Books.

Wachtel, A. (1989) "Child Abuse". Health & Welfare Canada Working Together: A 1989 National Forum on Family Violence, June 18-21.

Weedon, Chris (1987) *Feminist Practice & Poststructuralist Theory.* Oxford: Basil Blackwell.

Wiesel, Elie (1982) *Night.* New York: Bantam.

Williamson, Janice (1994) "Writing Aversion The Proliferation of Contemporary Canadian Women's Child Sexual Abuse Narratives" in Wendy Waring (ed.) *By, For & About: Feminist Cultural Politics.* Toronto: Women's Press.

Winnicott, D.W. (1990) *The Maturational Processes and the Facilitating Environment.* London: Karnac Books.

Wisechild, Louise (1988) *The Obisidian Mirror.* Seattle: Seal Press.

Wyckoff, Hogie (1980) *Solving Problems Together.* New York: Grove Press.

Young, Iris, (1990) *Justice & The Politics of Difference.* Princeton N.J.: Princeton University Press.

Acknowledgements

Writing appears to be a solitary activity. In practice, it requires support from those within the writer's community. I am very grateful for the knowledge, affection and encouragement of the following individuals within my life as well as this work:

Kari Dehli for pushing the theoretical edges of this work, and Kathleen Rockhill for her support of this project. Kate McKenna, Becky Anweiler and Ruth Goldman for their support through the early days.

Lynne Raskin, Marilyn Struthers, Kathleen Coleman, Gillian Lewis, Patrick Lewis for living beside me through the process with such affection.

The members of the writing group, Ann Decter, Tara Goldstein, Sharon Rosenberg, Jenny Horsman for their consistent encouragement, their ability to get me unstuck and the power of their direction to "say more".

Sharon Rosenberg whose engagement with me through intellectual discussion, emotional support and practical assistance is an invaluable gift.

Marilyn Vivian, whose affection and witnessing over time has brought my places of silence towards speech and created new possibilities within my life.

Ann Decter, whose wisdom and matter of fact approach to shaping this work encouraged my emerging voice and the development of this text.

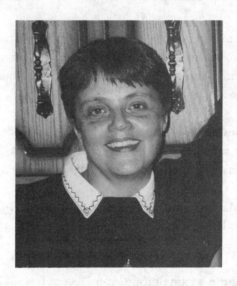

Tanya Lewis has a PhD. in Community Psychology from the Ontario Institute for Studies in Education at University of Toronto. She has worked in social services for many years. Tanya lives in Toronto with her two teenaged children and a needy cat. *Living Beside* is her first book.